GOVERNORS STATE UNIVERSITY LIBRARY

3 1611 00084 1590

7 W9-CPQ-957

Implications of the Americans with Disabilities Act for Psychology

Susanne M. Bruyère, PhD, CRC, is currently the Director of the Program on Employment and Disability in the School of Industrial and Labor Relations—Extension Division, and the Director/Senior Consultant of the Faculty /Health Program of University Human Resource Services at Cornell University. Dr. Bruyère has also served as the Project Director of the National Materials Development Project on the Employment provisions of the ADA, and Training Director of the Northeast Disability and Business Technical Assistance Center. Prior to her current position, she served as an Associate Professor in the Department of Rehabilitation and as Assistant Director in the Region X Rehabilitation Continuing Education Program at Seattle University. She received her doctoral degree in Rehabilitation Counseling Psychology from the University of Wisconsin—Madison, and has Master's degrees in Rehabilitation Counseling, Public Administration, and Adult Education. She is a Past President of the Division of Rehabilitation Psychology of the American Psychological Association, and President-Elect of the National Council on Rehabilitation Education. Dr. Bruyère is a Certified Rehabilitation Counselor and a Certified Special Educator.

Janet O'Keeffe, DrPH, is the Assistant Director for Public Interest Policy in the Public Policy Office of the American Psychological Association (APA), where she works on a wide range of health, aging, and disability issues. In that capacity, she participated in the effort to enact the Americans with Disabilities Act and worked specifically to ensure that persons with stigmatized disabilities such as AIDS and mental illness were covered by the Act. She currently co-chairs the Consortium for Citizens with Disabilities (CCD) Task Force on Health, and the CCD Task Force on Long-Term Services and Supports.

Dr. O'Keeffe received her Bachelor of Science in Nursing from the State University of New York and has worked as a Registered Nurse in a variety of health care settings, including hospitals, nursing homes, rehabilitation centers, ambulatory care and home care. She received her Master's and Doctorate degrees in Public Health from the UCLA School of Public Health. Prior to her position at APA, Dr. O'Keeffe was the Assistant Project Director for California Lt. Governor Leo McCarthy's Task Force on the Feminization of Poverty. She also worked as a Congressional Fellow in the U.S. House of Reepresentatives and as a legislative and policy analyst on long-term care and health personnel policy for the American Association of Retired Persons.

Implications of
the Americans with Disabilities Act
FOR PSYCHOLOGY

Susanne M. Bruyère, PhD, CRC
Janet O'Keeffe, DrPH

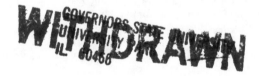

AMERICAN PSYCHOLOGICAL ASSOCIATION
Washington, DC

SPRINGER PUBLISHING COMPANY
New York

RM 930.5 .U6 I47 1994

Implications of the
Americans with Disabilities

3 1 2 7 20

Copyright © 1994 Springer Publishing Company, Inc.
and the American Psychological Association.

All rights reserved. No part of the book may be reproduced in any form, by photostat,
microform, retrieval system, or any other means, without the prior written permission
of the publisher.

American Psychological Association
750 First Street, NE
Washington, DC 20002

Springer Publishing Company, Inc.
536 Broadway
New York, NY 10012-3955

94 95 96 97 98 / 5 4 3 2 1

Cover and interior design by Holly Block
Production Editor, Pam Ritzer

Library of Congress Cataloging-in-Publication Data
Implications of the Americans with Disabilities Act for psychology /
  Susanne M. Bruyère, Janet O'Keeffe, editors.
      p.   cm.
  Originally published as companion special issues of *Consulting Psychology Journal* and
Rehabilitation Psychology.
      Includes bibliographical references and index.
        ISBN 0-8261-8450-2
        1. Rehabilitation—United States. 2. United States. Americans
with Disabilities Act of 1990. I. Bruyère, Susanne M.
II. O'Keeffe, Janet. III. Consulting Psychology Journal.
IV. Rehabilitation Psychology.
RM930.5.U6I47   1994
362.2'0973—dc20

                                                        93-39427
                                                        CIP

Printed in the United States of America

Contents

Contributors

Christopher G. Bell, Counsel
Jackson, Lewis, Schnitzler and Krupman
Washington, DC 20006

Susanne M. Bruyère, Ph.D., C.R.C.
Director, Program on Employment and Disability
Cornell University
School of Industrial and Labor Relations
Ithaca, NY 14853-3901

Paul J. Carling, Ph.D.
Executive Director
Center for Community Change, Institute for Program Development
Trinity College-McAuley Hall
Burlington, VT 05401-1496

Nancy M. Crewe, Ph.D.
Professor, Dept. of Counseling,
Education Psychology and Special Education
Michigan State University–College of Education
East Lansing, MI 48824-1034

Nancy L. Jones, J.D.
Legislative Attorney
Congressional Research Service, Law Division
Washington, DC 20540

Richard J. Klimoski, Ph.D.
Professor and Vice Chair
Dept. of Psychology
The Ohio State University–Townsend Hall
Columbus, OH 43210-1222

Mary Anne Nester, Ph.D.
Branch Chief for Professional & Administrative Examining
U.S. Office of Personnel Management
Washington, DC 20415

Janet O'Keeffe, Dr.P.H.
Assistant Director for Public Interest Policy
Public Policy Office
American Psychological Association
Washington, DC 20002-4242

Susan N. Palmer
Director of Corporate Relations
Kenan-Flagler Business School
University of North Carolina–Chapel Hill
Chapel Hill, NC 27599

Deborah A. Pape, Ph.D.
Vocational Rehabilitation Psychologist
Workers' Evaluation Rehabilitation Center
St. Mary's Medical Center
Racine, WI 53405

Cathy A. Redd, Ph.D.
Washington Crossing, PA 18977

Paul R. Sachs, Ph.D.
Professional Psychology Group
Bala Cynwyd, PA 19004

Vilia M. Tarvydas, Ph.D., C.R.C.
Assistant Professor and Coordinator
Rehabilitation Psychology Program
University of Iowa
Iowa City, IA 52242

Preface

Disability has become a major factor in the lives of all members of our society. It is a virtual certainty that one or more members of almost every American family will develop a disability at some point in their lives. Thus, disability has become a common characteristic of human experience. Currently, there are an estimated 43 million Americans with disabilities of all kinds and this figure is increasing rapidly as modern medical science enables more and more people to survive previously fatal birth defects, injuries, and illnesses, many times with severe and life-long impairments. The dramatic increase in the lifespan of persons with disabilities represents an historic enlargement of the human potential. Yet our culture has not yet modified its policies and practices to assist in the fulfillment of that potential.

In this regard, the Americans with Disabilities Act (ADA) is a landmark piece of legislation mandating not only that change our physical environment to accommodate persons with disabilities, but that we change our thoughts and attitudes about persons with disabilities. The ADA challenges our nation to end discrimination against persons with disabilities and to promote their participation in the productive mainstream society. When considering the importance of the ADA to our nation, it is important to remember that unlike other legislation prohibiting discrimination against a class of individuals, the ADA potentially applies to every American.

Because the ADA addresses all aspects of society and covers persons with many different types of disabilities, it is necessarily a complex piece of legislation. Given this, it is extremely important that those with responsibilities under the ADA understand how the law affects them, and determine what they need to do to comply with both the letter and the spirit of the law. This book on the ADA and psychology is a major contribution to that end. It is my hope that as more people become aware of the reasonable responsibilities imposed by the ADA, and the magnificent opportunities it offers, they will move from an attitude of fear and hesitation to one of enthusiastic support for its goal: a more just and productive society.

JUSTIN DART, PAST CHAIRMAN
THE PRESIDENT'S COMMITTEE ON EMPLOYMENT
OF PEOPLE WITH DISABILITIES

Editors' Introduction and Overview

Why a publication on the Americans with Disabilities Act (ADA)? The ADA is a landmark piece of civil rights legislation that extends the prohibition against discrimination on the basis of race, sex, religion, and national origin to persons with disabilities. Because the ADA covers all aspects of participation in society—employment, public accommodations, transportation, and telecommunication—its impact will be felt in multiple ways. Individuals may have both rights and responsibilities under the law according to the many different roles they assume: as employers or consultants to employers, as practitioners providing health services to the public, or as individuals who today, or in the future, may be protected by the Act. If the ADA is to be fully implemented, it is essential that those with rights and responsibilities under the Act be knowledgeable regarding its provisions. The provisions of the ADA have relevance to psychologists and other health care providers in terms of their practice, research, and training. Employers, human resource professionals, and labor union representatives also need to be apprised of the requirements of the ADA in order to respond appropriately to accommodation requests by workers with disabilities.

This book discusses the significance of the ADA for employers, human resource professionals, psychologists, and other health care providers, in such areas as assessment, reasonable accommodation considerations with special populations, new consulting opportunities, and training. The inclusion of authors from a variety of professional backgrounds and the range of issues covered underscore the need for an interdisciplinary effort to ensure implementation of the ADA. In order to fulfill their responsibilities under the ADA, health care professionals such as psychologists, rehabilitation counselors, and employee assistance professionals need to be aware, not only of those areas of disability law and policy that are relevant to their work, but also the resources that are available to facilitate compliance with the law. For this reason, we have included a resource list in a special Appendix to help ensure timely access to expert information and advice.

The first chapter discusses the prevalence of disability and discrimination, and provides a brief overview of the Act's definitions and central provisions. In subsequent chapters, these definitions and provisions are explored in more detail and analyzed from unique perspectives; each chapter stands alone as a reference on a particular issue. In the area of pre-employment screening, employers, human resource professionals, and psychologists need to be aware of the impact of the ADA on the administration of psychometric tests. The chapter by Mary Anne Nester, Branch Chief for Professional and Administrative Examining for the US Office of Personnel Management, addresses the legal and psychometric issues related to nondiscrimination in employment testing for persons who have disabilities. In a related chapter, Richard Klimoski and Susan Palmer review the ADA's potential impact on the recruitment and assessment of job applicants.

The ADA has implications for those individuals and organizations working with special populations regarding accommodations that may be requested as individuals seek reintegration into the workplace. Paul Sachs and Cathy Redd address the implications for individuals with neurological impairments with attention to prevocational assessment, vocational re-entry, and workplace adjustment. Paul Carling discusses reasonable accommodation issues for persons with psychiatric disabilities.

In many areas, the Americans with Disabilities Act may provide new opportunities for expanded practice and consultation for a variety of health care professionals. Chris Bell, former Director of the ADA Technical Assistance Unit of the Equal Employment Opportunity Commission and currently a consultant with Milt Wright and Associates, discusses the interplay between the workers' compensation system and the ADA, and its implications for rehabilitation professionals. The implications of the ADA for those providing services for individuals with alcohol and drug addictions are discussed in the chapter by Nancy Jones, Legislative Attorney with the Congressional Research Law Division of the Library of Congress.

The Americans with Disabilities Act has significant implications for the training of rehabilitation psychologists and other health care professionals. Nancy Crewe advises psychology programs about considerations that must be made in examining admissions criteria and procedures to avoid discrimination against applicants with disabilities. These considerations apply equally to other health profession programs. As discussed by Pape and Tarvydas, only a minority of psychologists have any specialized training in the area of disability or reasonable accommodation. These authors discuss the types of services that will be needed to support implementation of the ADA and its implications for the professional scope of practice of psychologists. Functional hierarchies for training based on a model of consultative practice are presented, including rehabilitation principles, knowledge and functions, disability concepts, and specific knowledge about the Americans with Disabilities Act. Resources for further reading in each of these areas are provided.

It is our hope that this information on specific areas related to psychology and the Americans with Disabilities Act contributes to your professional practice and interest in the development and enhancement of services to individuals with disabilities.

SUSANNE M. BRUYÈRE
DIRECTOR, PROGRAM ON EMPLOYMENT AND DISABILITY
SCHOOL OF INDUSTRIAL AND LABOR RELATIONS, CORNELL UNIVERSITY

JANET O'KEEFFE
ASSISTANT DIRECTOR FOR PUBLIC INTEREST POLICY
PUBLIC POLICY OFFICE, AMERICAN PSYCHOLOGICAL ASSOCIATION

·1·

Disability, Discrimination, and the Americans with Disabilities Act

Janet O'Keeffe

On July 26, 1990, the Americans with Disabilities Act (ADA) was signed into law. Many have called it the most significant piece of civil rights legislation since the passage of the 1964 Civil Rights Act which barred discrimination in employment, public accommodations and federally funded programs on the basis of race, sex, religion and national origin. By extending the same civil rights protections to persons with disabilities, the law mandates a policy of inclusion and fosters independence for the largest minority in the United States. As such, the ADA is likely to be the most important piece of legislation ever enacted for persons with disabilities.

Prevalence of Disability

For many people, the term disability brings to mind a picture of a person in a wheelchair. This is not surprising since mobility impairments are among the most immediately visible disabilities, and the international symbol for disability is a figure in a wheelchair. However, there are many other diseases and conditions that cause limitations in functioning and that can be disabling, though not all functional impairments result in disability. Rather, it is the interaction between an impairment and the social and physical environment that determines whether a specific impairment will, in fact, be disabling. Disability has been defined as "the expression of a physical or mental limitation in a social context—the gap between a person's capabilities and the demands of the environment" (Pope & Tarlov, 1991, p.1). Some of the conditions with a high probability of functional impairment include mental retardation, lung cancer,

1

multiple sclerosis, cerebral palsy, blindness, orthopedic impairments, rheumatoid arthritis, emphysema, and cerebrovascular disease (LaPlante, 1990). A review of all conditions causing impairment indicates that chronic diseases are increasingly a major cause of disability. There are several reasons for this trend.

Significant public health and medical advances in this century have led to a major increase in life expectancy. This is due in large part to decreases in the infant mortality rate, but also to decreases in age-specific mortality rates throughout the lifespan. Medical technology has enabled the survival of thousands of low birth weight babies and accident victims, many with severe disabilities. Many people are living longer, and as they age, develop chronic diseases and conditions which lead to significant impairments. Additionally, with advances in the treatment of infectious diseases, many more of those individuals with chronic diseases are living longer than they otherwise would have.

A recent report from the Institute of Medicine estimated that approximately 35 million Americans (one in seven) have disabling conditions that interfere with daily activities (Pope & Tarlov, 1991). Of the 11.3 million who are severely and chronically impaired, approximately 5.8 million are between the ages of 21 and 64, and approximately 4.5 million are over 65 (Center for Health Policy Development, 1992). Approximately 1.2 million have developmental disabilities, 1.5 million have severe and persistent mental illness, and 8.6 million have severe functional impairments due to physical causes (Center for Health Policy Development, 1992). Since the prevalence of chronic disease increases with age, as the "Baby Boom" cohort moves into middle-age and older, the coming decades will see an even larger increase in the number of persons with chronic impairments. Between 1970 and 1987, life expectancy in the U.S. increased by 4 years, but over half of this increase is time spent with activity limitations. Of the current 75-year life expectancy at birth, an average of 13 years will be spent with an activity limitation (Pope & Tarlov, 1991). This increasing prevalence of impairment and disability has been dubbed "the failure of success" (Gruenberg, 1977) and has led many health policy analysts to criticize the continuing emphasis in our medical research on saving life, rather than on preventing illness and ameliorating functional impairments.

Prevalence of Discrimination

Persons with disabilities are often excluded from the economic and social mainstream as a result of attitudinal, architectural, communications, and policy barriers. These barriers deny persons with disabilities the opportunity to access education, jobs, public accommodations and services, communications systems and public transportation, without which they cannot be independent, contributing members of society. They also impose major economic and social costs not only for the individual, but for society, through lost income tax revenues and the ever-escalating costs of dependency. In 1991 the U.S. spent $92 billion to assist persons with disabilities in meeting their basic living needs (Center for Health Policy Development, 1992). These costs could be significantly reduced if more persons with disabilities were employed, a goal shared by the majority of working-age persons with disabilities. In one survey of working-age persons with disabilities, although 78 percent stated they wanted to work, 66 percent were unemployed. Of these, 66 percent cited numerous barriers to doing so (Harris, 1986).

Persons with disabilities are disadvantaged on many measures. Approximately half of adults with disabilities have household incomes of $15,000 or less compared with 25 percent of persons without disabilities (U.S. Senate, 1989); and the poverty rate among persons with disabilities aged 16–64 is 28 percent compared to 9 percent for those without disabilities (Center for Health Policy Development, 1992).

Testimony presented to the Congress during enactment of the ADA highlighted the terrible toll of prejudice and discrimination on the lives of persons with disabilities. Witness after witness presented examples from their own experience of the insults and indignities they suffered because of their disabilities, as well as accounts of the many barriers which prevented them from participating in society. One woman who contracted polio as a child and uses a wheelchair, recounted how an attempt was made to remove her and a disabled friend from an auction house because they were "disgusting to look at" (U.S. House of Representatives, 1990, p. 29). Discrimination against persons with disabilities is often based on fear regarding the supposed effects of their disability on others. In one case, a woman with severe arthritis was denied a job because "college trustees [thought] that 'normal students shouldn't see her'" (Ibid. p. 30). In another instance, a New Jersey zoo refused admittance to a group of children with Downs Syndrome because it was feared they would "upset the chimpanzees" (Ibid. p. 30). Lack of protection from discrimination has reinforced and even fueled prejudice, particularly in the case of highly stigmatized conditions such as AIDS (U.S. Senate, 1989).

The harm caused by attitudinal barriers may be the most difficult to measure, but in many instances imposes the greatest individual cost when persons with disabilities internalize the experience of discrimination, leading to a sense of inadequacy and low self-esteem (West, 1991). Psychological research has demonstrated the pervasive nature of stigma associated with disabilities of all kinds (Asch, 1989). Stigmatized populations such as persons with disabilities are viewed by some as less than human and this perception is used to justify discriminatory treatment (Ibid.). Other negative attitudes supporting discriminatory treatment include: the perception of disability as punishment for moral transgression, the view that disabilities render persons helpless and dependent, and that persons with disabilities are incapable of full social and economic participation in society (Ibid.). Stigmatizing and discriminatory attitudes are particularly severe for persons with mental disabilities, especially those with serious, persistent mental illness and for persons with a history of alcohol and drug dependency, even after full recovery. Persons with these conditions are often considered responsible for their own illness, and frequently evoke judgmental attitudes.

Purpose and Essential Provisions of the ADA

The purpose of the ADA is "to provide a clear and comprehensive national mandate for the elimination of discrimination against individuals with disabilities and to provide clear, strong, consistent, enforceable standards addressing discrimination against individuals with disabilities."[1] The ADA prohibits discrimination against persons with disabilities by all private and public entities in the areas of employment, housing, transportation, telecommunications, and public accommodations and services operated by private entities.

The establishment of civil rights for persons with disabilities has a long legislative history. While many laws contributed to the establishment of these rights, the groundwork for the ADA was laid with the passage of two major pieces of civil rights legislation. First, Section 504 of the Rehabilitation Act of 1973, and subsequent amendments, prohibited discrimination against persons with disabilities by federal employers and entities receiving federal funds. Second, with the passage of the 1988 Fair Housing Act Amendments, civil rights protections for persons with disabilities were extended to cover the private sector in the area of housing. Many of the provisions in the ADA are similar or identical to those in Section 504 and the Fair Housing Act. Section 504 is perhaps most significant, since its implementation over a 17-year period helped to define the core concepts included in the ADA.

Definition of Disability

The ADA defines disability broadly as "a physical or mental impairment that substantially limits one or more (of the) major life activities; a record of such impairment; or being regarded as having such an impairment."[2] A major life activity includes such things as seeing, hearing, walking, caring for oneself, learning, breathing and working.[3] Regulations published by the Equal Employment Opportunity Commission (EEOC) clarify that in determining whether an impairment is "substantially limiting," it is important to examine the conditions, manner, or duration under which an activity can be performed in comparison to most people (1991).[4]

Other important factors to consider are an impairment's nature and severity, its duration, and its permanent or long-term impact.[5] The EEOC also states that "the existence of an impairment is to be determined without regard to mitigating measures such as medication, or assistive or prosthetic devices."[6] Thus, even if the symptoms of diabetes are totally controlled by the use of insulin, a person with diabetes is still considered to have an impairment. The definition of impairment does not include physical characteristics such as eye color and height which are within "normal" range and are not the result of a physiological disorder. Similarly, personality traits such as poor judgment and/or a quick temper are not considered an impairment unless they are symptoms of a mental or psychological condition such as retardation or traumatic brain injury, in which case they may be considered impairments.[7] The ADA's broad definition of disability was adopted to take account of the distinct features of a wide variety of disabling conditions as well as the numerous ways in which discrimination occurs.

A major distinction between disability and other protected categories, such as race and gender, is that a disability is not a fixed characteristic. People may recover totally from disabling conditions, or they may experience periods of recovery if they have a condition characterized by exacerbations and remissions, such as mental illness and multiple sclerosis. Thus, persons can be discriminated against on the basis of a history of disability, a situation frequently encountered by persons with a history of mental illness. This fact underlies the ADA's protection of persons with a "record of an impairment."

The inclusion of persons who are "regarded as" having an impairment in the ADA definition of disability demonstrates an understanding of the many different ways in which discrimination occurs. It recognizes that persons with physical or mental impairments, and persons with marked physical differences, may not, in fact, be disabled; but because of myths and stereotypes about their condition, or outright prejudice, may be denied access to employment, housing or public accommodations. Under this part of the definition, persons with disfigurements such as facial scarring and persons with malformed but fully functional limbs, who are discriminated against solely on the basis of their appearance, are protected.

There is also a provision in the ADA that protects persons who are discriminated against on the basis of an association or relationship with a person who has a known disability.[8] Such discrimination could occur for a variety of reasons. During Congressional hearings, a woman from Kentucky told how she had been fired from a job she had held for many years after her employer found out that she was taking care of her son who had AIDS (U.S. Senate, 1989). In another example, the EEOC ruled that if a job applicant states that his or her spouse has a disability and is then turned down because the employer believes the applicant will likely be absent from work to take care of the spouse, this person is also protected by the ADA.[9]

Qualified Individual with a Disability

A major concern expressed during enactment of the ADA and since passage is that the ADA is an affirmative action law that will lead to the hiring of unqualified persons simply because they have a disability. In fact, the ADA does not require affirmative action to increase the number of persons with disabilities in the workplace. The Act clearly states that a person must be qualified to perform the job in question, with or without a reasonable accommodation. For example, a person who is blind is clearly not qualified to be a proofreader since the essential function of the job is the ability to read. However, in another job, reading may be just one of many job functions and the disability may be accommodated in a number of ways, including having co-workers and supervisors rely on spoken rather than written communications, and/or providing a reader when required. A person with low vision could be provided with equipment which enlarges print. Similarly, persons with speech impairments may utilize electronic communications equipment or low technology letter/word boards to communicate. The House Committee on Education and Labor specifically stated in its report that the inclusion in the law of the term "qualified individual with a disability" affirms that the ADA "does not undermine an employer's ability to choose and maintain qualified workers" (U.S. House of Representatives, 1990). See Klimoski and Palmer (Chapter 4) for a fuller discussion of this issue and other issues related to the hiring of persons with disabilities.

Reasonable Accommodation

Discrimination against persons with disabilities has two aspects: prejudice and barriers. The latter is defined as "any aspect of the social or physical environment that prevents meaningful involvement by persons with disabilities" (West, 1991). The most obvious example is a building that is inaccessible to a person in a wheelchair because there is no ramp or elevator. Another is an emergency telephone service (911) without a telecommunications device (TDD) or relay services communication system for speech- and hearing-impaired individuals. It is these and other barriers to access that generate the requirement for reasonable accommodation that is found in the ADA.

The requirement to provide reasonable accommodations distinguishes the ADA from other civil rights legislation in that it requires covered entities to take some action to either remove a barrier or, particularly in the employment setting, to adapt the environment so that the person can function on a "level playing field." It is this requirement for "action" on the part of employers that may be responsible for the mistaken belief that the ADA requires affirmative action to ensure that the category of "persons with disabilities" is represented in the workforce.

Title III of the Act deals with public accommodations, and states that "no individual shall be discriminated against on the basis of disability in the full and equal enjoyment of the goods, services, facilities, privileges, advantages, or accommodations of any place of public accommodations by any person who owns, leases (or leases to), or operates a place of public accommodation."[10] Entities covered by the term "public accommodations" includes numerous facilities such as restaurants, hotels, theaters, museums, and the offices of health care providers.[11] Psychologists, as health care providers, are considered public accommodations and so may be required to comply with the ADA in a variety of ways. Health care providers may be required to provide auxiliary aids or services for persons seeking treatment, or to make architectural modifications to their office space. Such determinations are likely to be highly individualized and must be dealt with on a case-by-case basis. Specific situations, where it is not clear if there is an obligation under the law, will require consultation with an attorney knowledgeable about the ADA and related disability case law.

Since the ADA went into effect, the Justice Department, which is responsible for enforcement of the ADA's public accommodation provisions, has received over 1500 allegations of violations of the ADA and all were resolved without litigation. However, in 1992, the Department filed its first complaint against a company with over 10,000 students nationwide, for refusing to provide sign language interpreters or other aids necessary for hearing-impaired students to fully participate in their course. The course prepares accountants to take a national certified public accountant examination, which most states require before they can prepare tax documents for clients. In its suit, the Department alleges that the company violated two separate provisions of the ADA: one requiring that courses for professional certification be offered in a manner accessible to persons with disabilities, and another, which requires that private entities provide "auxiliary aids" when necessary to ensure effective communication. These aids include sign language interpreters, note takers, written transcripts, and other methods to enable hearing-impaired persons to access orally delivered materials.

During passage of the ADA and since enactment, concerns have been voiced regarding the financial burden of providing these types of reasonable accommodation provisions. However, the ADA states that entities covered by the public accommodations of Title III do not have to provide reasonable accommodations unless they are "readily achievable," and that employers covered under Title I do not have to provide reasonable accommodations if they constitute an "undue hardship."

Readily Achievable and Undue Hardship

The ADA defines "readily achievable" as "easily accomplishable and able to be carried out without much difficulty or expense."[12] Examples include the provision of some of the auxiliary aids cited above, and in the case of architectural barriers, the installation of ramps, grab bars, and lever handles to replace door knobs. Other accommodations could include the widening of doorways to ensure that customers or clients can enter a facility and use all of the amenities open to the public, including restrooms. The definition of "readily achievable" is measured by the same factors that are used to determine an "undue hardship." "Undue hardship" is defined as "an action which will require significant expense or difficulty, when considered in light of a variety of factors, including the nature and cost of the accommodation, the overall financial resources of the employer, the size of the business with respect to the number of employees, and the number, type, and location of its facilities."[13] This definition was further clarified by the EEOC in its ruling that a business would not have to alter its fundamental nature in order to accommodate a person with a disability. As an example, they noted that a dimly lit nightclub would not be required to install bright lights to accommodate a waiter with limited vision since it would fundamentally alter the ambience of the nightclub, and therefore, the nature of the business.[14] However, if the use of a flashlight would enable the person to work safely, this would be considered a reasonable accommodation. It is clear from the legislative history of the ADA that in terms of the level of effort required, Congress intended the "undue hardship" standard for employers to be a higher standard than that of "readily achievable" for public accommodations (Jones, 1991). Whether or not a reasonable accommodation is possible or acceptable in a given situation, it is important to document fully all efforts that are made to accommodate a person with a disability.

Concerns about the costs of providing reasonable accommodations were addressed by Congress through a change in the tax code. To ease the burden on small businesses, Congress added an "access credit" to the tax code allowing these businesses, a tax credit for one-half of the first $10,000 (over $250) of the eligible costs of complying with the ADA.[15] Because a tax credit is deducted from the tax owed, the cost of the accommodation is being borne by the federal government as revenue foregone, and is therefore spread broadly over society. The expenses for which the credit may be taken include the wide range of access expenditures recognized under the ADA as "auxiliary aids and services." These include interpreters for individuals with hearing impairments, readers and taped texts for individuals with visual impairments, and the acquisition or modification of equipment or devices (Schaffer, 1991). For the removal of physical barriers, both small and large businesses are allowed a tax deduction up to $15,000. To assist businesses in identifying appropriate accommodations, the President's Committee on Employment of People with Disabilities operates a Job Accommodation Network (JAN), which provides toll-free consultation to businesses regarding reasonable accommodations. Its success rate in providing assistance to businesses is 73 percent, and in 85 percent of its cases, the expense of making a modification to accommodate a person with a disability was less than $1,000 (President's Committee, 1992). For small businesses eligible for the tax credit, the cost of these accommodations would have been only $250 or less.

Areas of the ADA Needing Clarification

One of the major criticisms of the ADA is that its application in many potential situations is ambiguous and therefore open to widely different interpretations. This has caused some opponents of the Act to call it "The Lawyers' Employment Act." Supporters of the ADA respond by saying that every individual with a disability is unique and every situation involving barriers to inclusion is also unique. Thus, under the employment provisions, the Act can not require or guarantee a specific accommodation because a "case-by-case approach is essential if qualified persons of varying abilities are to receive equal opportunities to compete for an infinitely diverse range of jobs."[16] Rather, the ADA establishes parameters to guide employers in considering how to accommodate persons with disabilities. It is clear that certain situations and issues will probably have to be resolved in the courts, as they were with Section 504 of the Rehabilitation Act. Some of these ambiguities are to be expected in a law as comprehensive as the ADA. However, some of the ambiguities are a direct result of political and ideological conflicts that occurred during passage, most notably over the inclusion of persons with drug addictions.

Of particular concern for psychologists who treat persons with chemical dependencies is the provision which states that persons with drug addictions are protected by the ADA, only if they are in treatment and not illegally using drugs. Given that relapses during treatment are common, it is not clear how a court would rule if a person were fired from a job because of relapses over the course of treatment. A related question relates to recovery: when will a person be considered "recovered" from addiction? The report accompanying the Act clearly indicates that the limitations on the Act's protections are not to be narrowly construed to apply only to persons who use drugs "on the day of, or within a matter of weeks before, the action in question" (Jones, 1991). Thus, it is not clear whether a police department could be accused of discrimination for not hiring an applicant on the grounds that he or she had illegally used drugs in the previous month but was no longer using them (see Jones, Chapter 8, for a more detailed discussion). There is a need for more empirical research in this area to determine, with some degree of certainty, under what circumstances future drug use can be predicted based on past drug use, and the relationship between relapses and outcomes in drug treatment programs. The results of such research would likely be brought to bear in any legal proceedings regarding this issue. Another area of ambiguity relates to the use of psychological testing in employment settings. Still unresolved at the time of going to press is the question of whether such tests will be considered medical examinations under the ADA and therefore prohibited until after a conditional offer of employment has been made (see Klimoski and Palmer, Chapter 4).

Remaining Barriers

While the ADA is a comprehensive mandate to end discrimination against persons with disabilities, it does not address all of the barriers impeding their full participation in society. One important area that is not adequately addressed by the Act is the availability of health insurance. The inability of persons with disabilities to obtain adequate health insurance is a major barrier to their employment. A 1985 survey of persons with disabilities found that one of the most frequently cited barriers to employment was fear of losing government health benefits which are available to many persons with severe disabilities through the Medicare or Medicaid programs (Harris & Associates, 1985).

The current crisis in the U.S. health care system is felt most acutely by the millions of Americans with disabilities and chronic illnesses, and also by their families. The crisis in coverage is a direct result of the rapidly increasing costs of health care, which have led commercial insurers and employers who self-insure to engage in medical underwriting practices which exclude persons with chronic illnesses, persons with disabilities, and persons who are deemed at high risk of developing health conditions.

The issue of access to health insurance has been called by many the "missing piece" of the ADA. This was not an oversight, however, but a deliberate omission. The ADA specifically exempts insurance from its provisions, stating that nothing in the Act "shall be construed to prohibit or restrict an insurer, hospital or medical service company, health maintenance organization, or any agent or entity that administers benefit plans, or similar organizations from underwriting risks, classifying risks, or administering such risks that are based on or not inconsistent with State law."[17] However, the Act also states that nothing in the exemptions provided can be used as a subterfuge to evade the purposes of the Act, though it is not clear what exactly would constitute a subterfuge.[18]

While insurers are generally exempt from the provisions of the ADA, the Act does require that they use sound actuarial data to determine, classify, and rate risks. It is this provision which may be useful in challenging medical underwriting which is based solely on stereotypes or out-of-date, irrelevant data. For example, most insurers selling health, disability, long-term care, or life insurance deny coverage to persons with a history of mental health treatment. In the case of individuals with serious mental illness such as schizophrenia, there is research that indicates a higher risk of morbidity and mortality for these persons than for the general population. However, there are no extant data to support the rating of all persons who receive mental health treatment as high risk and "uninsurable." Despite this, insurers generally refuse to provide health, disability, or life insurance to any person who has received outpatient counseling or psychotherapy, even if such treatment was of brief duration and was terminated several years ago (O'Keeffe, 1992).

Anecdotal accounts of such practices have been reported to the National Mental Health Association, the Bazelon Center for Mental Health Law, and the American Psychological Association (Personal communications). In one case, a woman was denied coverage under her husband's employer's health policy because of her "mental health history," comprising four visits to a therapist to deal with adjustment problems related to the birth of her first child. In another case, a woman was told that seven visits to a therapist to deal with the severe illness of a family member would probably disqualify her from life insurance coverage, even though the therapy took place more than three years before. Persons who are aware of such practices often will not utilize their health insurance coverage for mental health treatment because they fear this type of future discrimination (Ibid.).

While the ADA exempts insurers from its provisions, except as noted above, the Act clearly covers the provision of employee benefits. Thus, an employer who is concerned about increases in health insurance premiums cannot deny employment to a qualified individual with a disability, or to an applicant who has a child with a disability, on these grounds (West, 1991). However, there is concern that due to the escalating costs of health insurance, this provision may well lead employers to either drop health insurance for all their employees or to fire or fail to hire persons with disabilities because of concerns about the cost of health insurance. Since the employment provisions of the law took effect on July 26, 1992, the EEOC has received 3,358 charges of discrimination under the ADA. Almost half were filed by persons alleging they were wrongly terminated from their jobs because of a disability or health condition (Disability Compliance Bulletin, 1993). The conditions most frequently represented include back disorders, mental illness, diabetes, heart impairments, visual and hearing impairments, alcoholism, epilepsy, arthritis, cancer, neurological impairments, and HIV infection (Ibid. p. 5). In a recent case in Minnesota, a woman with multiple sclerosis successfully sued her employer for purposely transferring her to a distant location to force her resignation and thereby avoid increased health insurance costs (Ibid. p. 12). Thus it is clear that while the ADA will not be able to assure access to health insurance, it can be an effective tool in reducing employment discrimination related to its provision.

In conclusion, the ADA has the potential to reduce and hopefully eliminate many forms of discrimination against persons with disabilities, but certainly not all. The realization of its mandate to end discrimination will require strong enforcement, the voluntary commitment and effort of millions of individuals, and the establishment of new policies to deal with issues that are not adequately addressed by the ADA.

Footnotes

1) 42 U.S.C. Sec. 12101
2) 42 U.S.C. Sec. 12102
3) 29 U.S.C. Sec. 706(8).
4) 29 C.F.R. 1630.2(h)(j).
5) 29 C.F.R. 1630.2(j)(2)(i-iii).
6) 28 C.F.R. 1630.2(h).
7) 29 C.F.R. 1630.2(h).
8) 29 C.F.R. 1630.8
9) 29 C.F.R. 1630.8
10) 42 U.S.C. Sec. 12182
11) 42 U.S.C. Sec. 12181
12) 42 U.S.C. Sec. 12182
13) 42 U.S.C. Sec. 12111.

14) 29 C.F.R. 1630.2(p).
15) Revenue Reconciliation Act of 1990, P.L.
    101-508, Sec. 11611 (a).
16) 29 C.F.R. 1630; Appendix.
17) 42 U.S.C. Sec. 12201 (c).
18) 42 U.S.C. Sec. 12201 (c)

References

Asch, A. (1984). The experience of disability: A challenge for psychologists. *American Psychologist, 39*(5), 529–536.

Center for Health Policy Development. (1992). *Familiar faces: The status of America's vulnerable populations: A chartbook.* Portland, ME: Author.

Disability Compliance Bulletin. (February 3, 1993). Transfer of employee was designed to force resignation. Author, 3(14). Horsham, PA: LRP Publications.

Equal Employment Opportunity Commission. (July 26, 1991). 29 CFR Part 1630. *Equal employment opportunity for individuals with disabilities; Final Rule.*

Jones, N. L. (1991) Essential requirements of the Act: A short history and overview. In J. West (Ed.), *The Americans with Disabilities Act: From policy to practice.* NY: Milbank Memorial Fund.

Gruenberg, E.M. (1977). The failures of success. *Milbank Memorial Fund Quarterly: Health and Society,* 55(3), 3-24.

Harris, L., & Associates. (1986). *Disabled Americans' self-perceptions: Bringing disabled Americans into the mainstream.* A survey conducted for the International Center for the Disabled. New York.

LaPlante, M.P. (1990). Disability risks of chronic illnesses and impairments. *Disability Statistics Report No.2.* Washington: National Institute on Disability and Rehabilitation Research.

O'Keeffe, J. (1992, Spring). Health care financing: How much reform is needed. *Issues in Science and Technology,* 42-49.

Pope, A.M., & Tarlov, A.R. (Eds.). (1991). *Disability in America: Toward a national agenda for prevention.* Washington: National Academy Press.

President's Committee on Employment of People with Disabilities. (August 1992). *Ready, willing and available: A business guide for hiring people with disabilities.* Washington, D.C.: Author.

Schaffer, Daniel C. (1991). Tax incentives. In J. West (Ed.), *The Americans with Disabilities Act: From policy to practice.* NY: Milbank Memorial Fund.

U.S. House of Representatives. (May 15, 1990). *Americans with Disabilities Act of 1990.* Report from the Committee on Education and Labor, No. 101-485, Part 2, to accompany H.R. 2273.

U.S. Senate. (August 30, 1989). *Americans with Disabilities Act of 1989.* Report from the Committee on Labor and Human Resources, No. 101-116, to accompany S. 933.

West, Jane. (1991). The social and policy context of the Act. In J. West (Ed.), *The Americans with Disabilities Act: From policy to practice.* NY: Milbank Memorial Fund.

· 2 ·

Implications of the Americans with Disabilities Act for the Training of Psychologists

Nancy M. Crewe

Passage of the Americans with Disabilities Act (ADA) has precipitated questions and some concerns for faculty in graduate psychology programs. For example, one program director acknowledged that he and his colleagues were quite upset by the prospect that they might be required by this new legislation to admit persons with schizophrenia into doctoral programs.

This chapter will address two issues. One, inherent in the concern just mentioned, are the ramifications of the ADA for the operation of University programs that train professional psychologists. The second is the kind of knowledge related to the ADA that needs to be incorporated into the education of psychologists who will be providing services to individuals with disabilities or who will be serving as consultants on this subject to employers or others.

The ADA and Admission to Graduate Psychology Programs

Beginning with the question that was raised by the program director, what does the ADA mean for doctoral and master's degree programs in Counseling, Clinical, Industrial, Organizational, and School Psychology? To some degree, the question comes 20 years late. The Rehabilitation Act of 1973 mandated nondiscrimination in programs receiving federal funding, either directly or through subcontracts, and this includes virtually all universities, both public and private in the United States. As a result, the settings in which psychologists work should have resolved problems of physical and programmatic access long ago. This includes a thorough

15

examination of admissions criteria and provision of accommodations to aid students with disabilities in accomplishing their academic goals.

The ADA, however, has brought new visibility to the struggle for equal access. Many psychology professors may have been unaware of the Rehabilitation Act, and others may have ignored it as a specialized piece of legislation that was not directly relevant to programs outside of the rehabilitation field. The ADA, on the other hand, explicitly addresses the whole spectrum of society, both public and private sectors. Now, even units that have had little experience with students who have disabilities are becoming more aware of their obligations to make their offerings accessible. It seems there has been far more media attention to the ADA than to previous legislation, so consumers have become more aware of their rights and more alert to barriers that stand in the way of their admission to and success within programs. They are starting to push for their rights under the ADA, thus raising awareness levels throughout society.

The ADA has major titles addressing employment, public services and transportation, public accommodations, and telecommunications. Education is not a separate title, in part because it has been covered by other legislation. Nevertheless, two provisions of the ADA that seem particularly relevant to training programs in psychology (and other disciplines as well) deserve special attention. One provision within Title III of the ADA requires access to public accommodations of many kinds including places of education—from nursery schools all the way through postgraduate programs. It prohibits "imposing or applying eligibility criteria that screen out or tend to screen out individuals with disabilities from fully and equally enjoying any goods, services, facilities, privileges, advantages, or accommodations unless such criteria can be shown to be necessary for the provision of the goods, services, facilities, privileges, advantages, or accommodations being offered" (Beck, 1992, p. 11). In addition, the ADA mandates that "examinations and courses, which often serve as gateways to employment and career advancement, must be fully accessible" (Benshoff, 1993, p. 129).

Under these provisions, programs are required to ensure that any admissions tests or other admissions criteria would not tend to screen out individuals with disabilities unless those measures bear directly on the person's ability to carry out the essential functions of a psychologist. The next challenge becomes that of defining the essential functions. In contrast to an employment situation where an applicant's qualifications can be compared to the demands of a specific position, evaluating the qualities that are essential requirements for a whole profession is most difficult. The actual activities and responsibilities of a psychologist in one setting (for example, a hospital) might be substantially different from that of a psychologist in another setting (say, a psychology department in a college of liberal arts), even if both are formally trained and identified as members of the same specialty area.

The American Psychological Association does not specify the admissions standards that programs should use in selecting students, although programs are asked to describe their criteria as part of the accreditation review. In the author's experience with admissions, some objective measures such as undergraduate or master's level grades, completion of specific courses and scores on the Graduate Record Examination are combined with more subjective criteria such as interpersonal skills, motivation, and reliability which may be reflected in letters of recommendation or interviews.

The validity of any of these criteria, particularly the more subjective ones, may be called into question. They might be defended on the basis of a consensus among academicians, but agreement would not rule out the possibility that the criteria are subject to attitudinal and other biases.

One possible source of data regarding the demands of applied psychology is the *Dictionary of Occupational Titles* (1991) and its related volume, *The Classification of Jobs According to Worker Trait Factors* (Field & Field, 1980). The latter publication reproduces Department of Labor data on the levels of ability needed to perform at a satisfactory (average) level in various occupations. Since the ratings for clinical, counseling, industrial, and school psychologists are very similar, they will be discussed as a group.

From the standpoint of physical strength, these occupations are minimally demanding, although all are said to require the ability to talk and hear, and all except counseling psychology also require the ability to see. (The rationale for distinctions among the subspecialties is not always apparent.) In terms of Reasoning Development, they are all rated at a level of 6 on a 6-point scale, indicating that the psychologist must

"Apply principles of logical or scientific thinking to a wide range of intellectual and practical problems. Deal with nonverbal symbolism (formulas, scientific equations, graphs, musical notes, etc.) in its most difficult phases. Deal with a variety of abstract and concrete variables. Apprehend the most abstruse class of concepts."

The requirement for mathematical development is generally rated at a level of 5, although industrial psychologists are rated as 6. The difference between those levels is a matter of degree, because both levels are described in the same way, as follows:

"Apply knowledge of advanced mathematical and statistical techniques such as differential and integral calculus, factor analysis, and probability determination, or work with a wide variety of theoretical mathematical concepts and make original applications of mathematical procedures, as in empirical and differential equations."

Language development is also demanded at a very high level (a rating of 6 for clinical psychologists and 5 for the others). This reflects:

Comprehension and expression of a level to

—Report, write, or edit articles for such publications as newspapers, magazines, and technical or scientific journals.

—Prepare and deliver lectures.

—Interview, counsel, or advise such people as students, clients, or patients in such matters as welfare eligibility, vocational rehabilitation, mental hygiene, or marital relations.

In terms of specific aptitudes, the ratings indicate that psychologists in all four specialties need to possess intelligence and verbal abilities in the top 10% of the population. Numerical ability needs to be in the top third for industrial and school psychologists and in the middle third for those in clinical and counseling areas. The other aptitude requirements (spatial, form, and clerical perception, motor coordination, finger and manual dexterity, eye/hand/foot coordination, and color discrimination) are set at the middle third of the population or lower.

The D.O.T. also describes interests and temperaments appropriate to occupations, so these might also form defensible bases upon which to select applicants. Interests in people and ideas, social and helping tasks, and prestige and esteem are common to most of the specialties, and clinical psychology is also high on interest in science and technology. In terms of temperaments, the following are noted for all or most of the areas: varied duties, dealing with people, influencing others, and subjective as well as objective evaluation of information.

Although these ratings provide some basis for determining characteristics that would serve as appropriate bases for admissions decisions, they are generalizations that could be interpreted quite differently from one university to another. Even something as straightforward as the ability to see and hear, for example, is not an invariable requirement for psychologists. While psychologists who have those abilities do utilize them in the course of work, some individuals who are blind or deaf also are effective psychologists. It seems reasonable to infer that the ADA (and other relevant legislation such as the Rehabilitation Act) would serve to place the burden of proof on the institution, requiring it to demonstrate that the criteria being used for admission are necessary and appropriate with respect to the ability to succeed in the training program and in the profession. Further, reasonable accommodations would need to be made for students whose functional limitations impede the learning process.

Accommodating Students with Disabilities in Psychology Programs

The easiest of the potential barriers to recognize and remediate are probably those involving physical limitations. The individual with motor weakness, for example, may need extra time or the assistance of another person to complete the Graduate Record Examination. Although some might question the appropriateness of modifying a standardized test, the Educational Testing Service has undertaken large-scale studies that provided data on the comparability of results when accommodations are made in the testing process for individuals with disabilities (Nester, 1993). Similarly, accommodations can generally be made with little difficulty for course examinations and even comprehensives within the training program itself because the faculty primarily want to determine whether the student has mastered the material rather than to know how quickly he or she can reproduce it.

More difficult questions arise in other areas including cognitive, communication, and emotional disabilities. Because they come closer to impinging on essential functions and responsibilities of a psychologist, it is not always clear whether accommodations within a training program are appropriate. Returning to the admissions process, consider the situation of a general (as opposed to rehabilitation) psychology program that typically includes interviews. Further, suppose that the candidate has a communication disability. Perhaps she has cerebral palsy and uses a communication board to express herself. The interview may be slow and uncomfortable for the faculty member conducting it, and this could reduce the candidate's chances of selection. Or the applicant might be deaf, leading to the use of an interpreter in the interview. Could this inhibit the applicant's freedom of expression or the interviewer's willingness to ask critical questions? And if these communication barriers do reduce the likelihood of admission, wouldn't that be a legitimate reflection of the problems the candidate will encounter in the practice of psychology since it involves substantial interpersonal communication?

Achieving equal access is even more difficult for individuals with disabilities involving cognitive or emotional impairments. Consider the following applicants:

(a) An individual who is highly intelligent but whose learning disabilities make it virtually impossible for him to organize coherent papers and essay examinations.

(b) A person whose traumatic brain injury has not impaired new learning but who has difficulty with impulse control and judgment in stressful situations.

(c) An individual who is an excellent student and a talented counselor but whose recurrent bouts of severe depression intermit-
tently interfere with her ability to work or study.

It is easier to ask these questions than to answer them, and since the
implementation of the ADA will rely heavily on the adjudication of individual cases, it is probably appropriate to leave the questions open.
However, it is essential for training directors to begin grappling with these
issues in order to clarify their own values and usual practices. It will not be
sufficient to rely upon assumptions about what "everybody knows" psychologists must be like. Such assumptions are frequently the basis for prej-
udicial patterns that the ADA was created to eradicate. For example, the
blind psychotherapist may be unable to see nonverbal responses, but she
may be fully as effective a communicator as one who is sighted.

Speaking as the director of a graduate program that has been vigorous
in recruiting and supporting students with varied disabilities, the author
admits that the right decisions are not always obvious. In general, we
have had minimal difficulties providing accommodations for a variety of
physical and sensory disabilities. Our success with persons who have
cognitive and emotional disabilities, on the other hand, has been mixed.
University programs are responsible, not only to the applicants and students in the program, but also to the clients who will some day depend
upon them for services. Graduates are eligible for state licensure, and the
program does bear a significant responsibility as a gatekeeper for that
credential. If the society is to be well served by the ADA, it will be important that when training programs take risks in admitting and accommodating students, that they also be allowed to exercise judgment about
when the student's performance fails to meet appropriate standards of
quality. This may sometimes lead to the difficult decision to terminate the
student. Cole and Lewis (1993) have summarized court cases that are relevant to the termination of social work trainees. They also provide guidelines for academic and disciplinary dismissals which should prove
extremely helpful to faculty members who struggle with making these
decisions validly and with fairness to all.

The ADA and the Psychology Curriculum

The ADA also has implications for the content of psychological training,
including some coursework that should be part of doctoral study for all
students in the various applied psychology programs. With the passage
of this act, individuals with disabilities were recognized more clearly
than ever before as members of a sociopolitical minority group.
Accordingly, content related to persons with disabilities should be inter-

woven throughout the curriculum in the same way as material concerning racial and ethnic minorities. For example, courses in social psychology should address negative attitudes toward persons with disabilities and the impact of bias on their interpersonal relationships and their opportunities for education, employment, housing, etc. Courses in psychological assessment should consider the need for reasonable accommodations in testing and the appropriateness of alternative approaches such as functional or situational assessment with this population. Interviewing courses should prepare students to interact in a facilitative manner with individuals who have various disabilities to reduce the potential interaction strain and to enhance the likelihood of developing a therapeutic relationship. If the program offers a special course in multicultural psychology, persons with disabilities should be discussed along with other diverse groups. As an aside, these lessons are more apt to be effective if they are learned in an integrated program. When students can develop peer relationships with classmates who have disabilities, they are much more likely to become comfortable enough to work well with such clients.

Psychologists who are planning to work as rehabilitation psychologists, of course, require considerably more specialized education related to disability and rehabilitation, and in-depth exposure to the ADA would constitute part of the curriculum. At the present time, the pattern of preparation in rehabilitation psychology varies widely from one institution to another. It is sometimes an independent doctoral specialization, sometimes a track within a clinical or counseling psychology program, and sometimes a postdoctoral program. Coursework may be tailored to psychology graduate students or it may be shared with students in other disciplines such as rehabilitation counseling or medical rehabilitation fields. Even in programs with a rich array of specialized courses, it seems unlikely that a whole course in a predoctoral program would be devoted to a single piece of legislation, but the ADA may be a focal point in a broader course on public policy, legislation, and the history of rehabilitation. It would also be likely to appear within courses on psychosocial aspects of disability, vocational assessment, job placement, consultation, and/or disability management.

For psychologists who are finished with their doctoral training and who desire to engage in consultative activities related to the ADA, continuing education of an extensive nature is indicated, particularly for those who do not have a strong existing background in disability and rehabilitation. Pape and Tarvydas (Chapter 9) developed a hierarchical model of training for such a practice. The first level involves an understanding of rehabilitation principles, knowledge, and functions including such areas as team facilitation, participation in advocacy groups, and application of rehabilitation legislation to practice. The second level involves mastery of disability concepts, functions, and knowledge, including, for example, knowledge of functional limitations related to various disabling conditions and the effective provision of various psychological services to such individuals. The third level focuses on the ADA knowledge and functions. They rightly emphasize that consultation regarding the ADA cannot be done well and ethically without a solid grounding in the psychology of disability and rehabilitation and without specific expertise in the particular area of disability that is being considered; for example, in mental retardation, psychiatric disabilities, or disabilities resulting from traumatic brain injury. Short-term training in the law itself will not provide the foundation necessary to apply it to the widely varied individuals and situations that will be encountered.

In summary, instruction on the ADA and its implementation needs to be brought into the predoctoral curriculum for all applied psychologists in the United States, not only for rehabilitation psychologists. For both practical and strategic reasons, this ought not to take the form of free standing courses on the ADA. Universities are continually fighting to hold the line against curriculum expansion that would further extend the time students must invest in obtaining their degrees. Students also resist adding courses to their lengthy programs. A possible exception might be students who are majoring in rehabilitation psychology or rehabilitation counselor education. The more effective alternative will be infusion and inclusion of an ADA perspective in a range of courses in the predoctoral curriculum. This approach will have the potential to reach a broader range of new professionals, not just specialists.

Different issues arise in the spheres of postdoctoral and continuing education. Within any of the formal postdoctoral programs in rehabilitation psychology, a specialized ADA course could be both appropriate and feasible. The curriculum development process is generally far more flexible than in predoctoral programs, and students are more amenable to advanced and specialized topics. With respect to continuing education, short-term, highly focused offerings are the rule. The challenge in this arena will be to avoid producing an army of "weekend experts" who have been exposed to the technicalities of the ADA and who go on to sell that knowledge without having proper grounding to do legitimate consultation. The ADA is a powerful piece of legislation that is highly relevant to psychologists. It is important that we provide opportunities for students and practitioners to understand it so that our field becomes a major contributor to its implementation.

Acknowledgments

This chapter was developed from a presentation provided at the American Psychological Association 1993 Annual Conference held in Toronto, for a special issue of *Rehabilitation Education*, focused on the implication of the Americans with Disabilities Act for rehabilitation education and training. The author would like to acknowledge the National Council on Rehabilitation Education for their willingness to allow use of this manuscript in this publication.

References

Beck, R. (1992). Working principles in the Americans with Disabilities Act (ADA). In J. K. O'Brien (Ed.), *National Short-Term Training Program: Americans with Disabilities Act*. Carbondale, IL: Southern Illinois University.

Benshoff, J. J. (1992). Accessibility issues, employment opportunities, and public accommodations. In J. K. O'Brien (Ed.), *National Short-Term Training Program: Americans with Disabilities Act*. Carbondale, IL: Southern Illinois University.

Cole, B. S., & Lewis, R. G. (1993). Gatekeeping through termination of unsuitable social work students: Legal issues and guidelines. *Journal of Social Work Education, 29*, 150–159.

Field, T. F., & Field, J. E. (1980). *The classification of jobs according to worker trait factors*. Roswell, GA: VDARE Service Bureau, Inc.

Nester, M.A. (1993). Psychometric testing and reasonable accommodation for persons with disabilities. *Rehabilitation Psychology, 38*, 75–85.

Pape, D. A., & Tarvydas, V. M. (1993). Responsible and responsive rehabilitation consultation on the ADA: The importance of training for psychologists. *Rehabilitation Psychology, 38*, 117–131.

U. S. Department of Labor, Manpower Administration (1977). *Dictionary of occupational titles*. Washington, DC: U.S. Government Printing Office.

· 3 ·

Psychometric Testing and Reasonable Accommodation for Persons with Disabilities

Mary Anne Nester

Federal laws and regulations of the last two decades have introduced the concept of nondiscrimination against persons with disabilities in the field of employment testing. The Rehabilitation Act of 1973, as amended, was the first far-reaching nondiscrimination law for disabled persons (29 U.S.C. 701-796i). Section 504 (29 U.S.C. 794) of that Act called for nondiscrimination by recipients of federal grants and, in the 1978 amendments, by the federal government. The regulations that were issued in the implementation of that Act introduced the requirement for reasonable accommodation to the physical or mental limitations of disabled persons, including the "appropriate adjustment or modification of examinations." The Americans with Disabilities Act (ADA) of 1990 (P.L. 101-336) extended the nondiscrimination protections to the entire private sector of the national economy. The ADA itself contained much of the language used in earlier regulations, including the requirement for reasonable accommodation and the inclusion of modified examinations as a form of accommodation.

Legal and Regulatory Requirements

The original Section 504 regulations (U.S. Department of Health, Education, and Welfare, 1977) spelled out the requirements for employment tests. They stated that employment criteria which screen out people with disabilities could not be used unless:

(1) the selection criterion had been shown to be job-related for the

25

position in question; (2) and there was no available job-related alternative that had less screen-out effect.

This wording has some similarity to the concepts of the Uniform Guidelines on Employee Selection Procedures (29 CFR 1607), but it does not contain the idea of a statistical showing of adverse impact. Undoubtedly, the writers of these regulations realized that the numbers of people with specific disabilities would be too small to permit such analyses. It should be noted that the Uniform Guidelines do not apply to enforcement of the Rehabilitation Act or the ADA.

The ADA requirements for selection criteria are specified in the Act itself and in the regulations to implement Title I of the Act (Equal Employment Opportunity Commission, 1991). Under the ADA, it is discriminatory to use a selection criterion that screens out individuals with disabilities unless the criterion is shown to be job-related for the position in question and is consistent with business necessity. The interpretive guidance for the regulations explains that the purpose of this provision is to ensure that tests do not act as barriers to the employment of persons with disabilities unless the person is unable to do the job, even with reasonable accommodation.

The EEOC regulations spell out additional requirements for the use of tests which, once again, are very similar to the regulations for the Rehabilitation Act. Paragraph 1630.11 of the regulation states:

It is unlawful for a covered entity to fail to select and administer tests concerning employment in the most effective manner to ensure that, when a test is administered to a job applicant or employee who has a disability that impairs sensory, manual, or speaking skills, the test results accurately reflect the skills, aptitude, or whatever other factor of the applicant or employee that the test purports to measure, rather than the impaired sensory, manual, or speaking skills of such employee or applicant (except where such skills are the factors that the test purports to measure).

In the interpretive guidance for this paragraph, it is explained that tests should not be given in formats that require use of the impaired skill, unless it is a job-related skill that the test is intended to measure.

Psychometric Context

The issue of nondiscrimination against persons with disabilities is a very new one in mainstream psychometrics and industrial/organizational psychology. Very little research has been devoted to it. Past research has focused on assessment for placement in educational, vocational, or rehabilitative settings, which have not involved the element of competition with persons who do not have disabilities. Therefore, there has not been much interest in establishing comparability of scores for persons with disabilities.

Research by Government Agencies

The U.S. Office of Personnel Management (OPM, formerly the U.S. Civil Service Commission) has had an interest in issues pertaining to testing persons with disabilities since approximately 1950. OPM develops tests and other instruments used to select people for jobs in the federal government. Applicants for these jobs are ranked on the basis of their test scores, and a selecting official must choose from the top three applicants on the rank-ordered list. In view of this highly competitive framework, OPM researchers have had to address the question of how to test applicants with disabilities so they can be ranked appropriately in terms of the characteristics the examinations are intended to assess.

The Panel on Testing Handicapped People

There has been a concern among psychometricians and others that the legal and regulatory requirements for testing disabled persons go beyond the state of the science in testing. This concern was addressed by a Panel on Testing Handicapped People, established at the National Academy of Sciences in 1979 under the sponsorship of the Office of Civil Rights in the Department of Education. In its final report (Sherman & Anderson, 1982), the panel concluded that contemporary practices in testing people with disabilities for employment and postsecondary school admission did not comply fully with federal antidiscrimination regulations. The panel recommended that programs of research be undertaken to validate tests for persons with disabilities through criterion-related studies.

APA Testing Standards

The issuance of the Standards for Educational and Psychological Testing (American Educational Research Association, American Psychological Association, and National Council on Measurement in Education, 1985) was a milestone because, for the first time, the standards included a chapter on "Testing People Who Have Handicapping Conditions." The chapter stressed that caution must be exercised in interpreting the validity of modified tests because of the lack of data about modified tests. However, the chapter encouraged the development of tests for persons with disabling conditions.

The concern about the validity of testing individuals with disabilities stems in part from the fact that nonstandard procedures must often be used. This requirement defies a basic principle of measurement: that standard procedures must be used and that departure from these procedures affects the measurement in an unknown way. Thus, even the most minor change, such as administering a vocabulary test in braille rather than in print, could potentially cast doubt on the validity of the test.

A related source of concern has been the issue of whether test scores from nonstandard administrations of standardized tests should be "flagged" to indicate the nonstandard administration. When scores on admissions or selection tests are flagged, selecting officials are alerted to the fact that the applicant has a disability. Pre-employment and pre-admission inquiry about disability is specifically prohibited by federal regulations, and flagging would seem to be a violation of the prohibition. However, if the test developers do not have a basis for believing that the results of the nonstandard testing have the same meaning as the results of standard testing, they are justified in using flagging to indicate their lack of confidence in the test results. This issue is discussed fully by Sherman and Anderson (1982).

The necessity of a research base for understanding the reliability and validity of accommodated testing was emphasized in Sherman and Anderson (1982) and in the 1985 testing standards. Fortunately, a massive series of studies carried out by the Educational Testing Service (ETS) in recent years has provided an excellent beginning for that research base.

ETS Studies

From 1982 through 1986, ETS conducted a series of integrated studies of the performance of test-takers with four types of disabilities — hearing impairment, learning disabilities, physical impairment, and visual impairment — on the Scholastic Aptitude Test (SAT) and the Graduate Record Examination (GRE) General Test. The results were described comprehensively in a book by Willingham, Ragosta, Bennett, Braun, Rock, and Power (1988).

The strategy of the ETS research was to assess the comparability of nonstandard and standard test scores using eight indicators of comparability: reliability, factor structure, differential item functioning, prediction of academic performance, admissions decisions, test content, satisfaction with testing accommodations, and test timing. To summarize broadly, Willingham et al. (1988) concluded that, "With the exception of test timing, these results indicate that the nonstandard versions of the SAT and GRE administered to handicapped examinees are generally comparable to the standard test in most important respects" (p. xiii). Some of their specific findings will be referred to later in this chapter. The wealth and uniqueness of the information presented by Willingham et al. make their book required reading for professionals interested in competitive testing issues. The ETS research is significant because it demonstrates that carefully thought-out test accommodations can be successful in preserving the reliability and validity of tests.

Types of Testing Accommodations

Testing accommodations will be discussed under three broad categories: testing medium, time limits, and test content. The interpretive guidance for EEOC's regulations for Title I of the ADA mentions all these categories as appropriate.

Testing Medium

A change in testing medium refers to the use of a different medium or method to present the same information. In most testing in this country, test information is presented in the English language. Therefore, braille, large print, reader, and audiotape are simply different ways (or modes or formats, as the EEOC's regulations call them) for presenting the same information. In most cases, these media could be interchanged without a change in the question content or the ability being tested. However, several problem areas exist in the use of different media:

1) Long reading passages may be more difficult when presented orally or in other media for visually impaired applicants. (In the ETS studies, visually impaired test-takers had complaints about long reading passages. However, their test scores do not appear to have been affected by this factor.)

2) Figural material is problematic. The embossing of figural material should not be viewed as a simple medium change, because the tactual sense is quite different from the visual sense (hence, the need for braille).

3) When readers are used, they should be people who read well and articulate clearly, and they should practice reading the test in advance. They should be warned against inadvertently giving clues to the test-taker when they read. A guide for examiners published by OPM (Heaton, Nelson, & Nester, 1980) contains suggestions for reading multiple-choice tests to applicants.

It should be noted that changing a test from a printed version into a sign language version is a translation into another language, rather than simply a change of medium. It must be done with all the care that would be taken in translating a test from English into, say, Japanese. (See Nester, 1984, for a discussion of this issue.)

Time Limits

In most cases of accommodated testing, it is necessary to change the test's time limits. Often the change in time limits causes a problem in interpreting test results. This problem arises because of the use of speeded power tests.

A pure power test is a test in which everyone has an opportunity to attempt to answer every question, and the scores are based on how many questions people can answer rather than on how fast they can work (see Nunnally, 1978, for a discussion of test time limits). The pure speed test, on the other hand, contains questions of trivial difficulty given with a very short time limit. Scores are based only on how fast people can work. Many tests intended to be power tests are actually somewhat speeded because a considerable number of people are unable to attempt every question. On a speeded power test, a person who had unlimited time would have an advantage over people who took it with the regular time limit. However, since many people with disabilities (e.g., braille-users) need extra time to take tests, there is the difficult problem of determining exactly how much extra time should be allotted so that the disabled test-taker is neither advantaged nor disadvantaged.

The ideal solution to this problem would be to eliminate the use of speeded power tests. Anyone who is in a position to make policy with respect to test time limits should argue for the use of very liberal time limits, with a completion rate of 90–95% of all test-takers. For such tests, disabled test-takers could be given unlimited time without having an undue advantage.

In the case of existing speeded power tests in which regular time limits cannot be changed, unlimited time may be inappropriate. ETS researchers, for example, concluded that the validity of the SAT for predicting freshman grades was impaired by the use of unlimited test time. They found a pattern of overprediction of grades for test-takers who received considerably extended test time, especially in the learning disabled group (Willingham et al., 1988).

One method of determining appropriate time limits is to conduct empirical studies, as recommended in the Standards for Educational and Psychological Tests. OPM conducted an empirical study to set time limits for visually impaired and deaf applicants on PACE (Nester, 1984). It was found that at least double time was needed for visually impaired users of all media to answer questions that consisted of a short reading passage followed by five answer choices. Mathematical questions involving computation required considerably more time than that. Such empirical studies are only possible in large-scale programs in which there are many test-takers. This is an area of research in which cooperative studies could be very fruitful.

Pure speed tests are used in the employment context to test such skills as perceptual speed and clerical checking. Such tests are clearly inappropriate for use with visually impaired test-takers because all the media for transmitting information are slower, and for physically impaired applicants because the physical mechanism for responding (e.g., marking the answer sheet) is slower. The time limit cannot be adjusted on these tests because speed is the factor that is being tested. Therefore, such tests must sometimes be eliminated from a test battery. This would be an instance of the last type of test accommodation — change of test content.

Test content

In the context of competitive testing for persons with disabilities, changes in test content are not made frequently. However, it is clear that this type of change is a form of accommodation that may be required for compliance with the ADA. From the standpoint of industrial/organizational psychology, any change in test content would need to be consistent with the validity strategy on which the test was based. For example, substituting one test question for another is easily done under a construct validity model, but might be troublesome under a content validity model.

Changes in test content can be divided for convenience into three types: change in individual test questions, change in the question type, and change or deletion of a knowledge, skill, or ability (KSA) that is being measured. The first type of change, as mentioned above, is easily done in a construct-valid test. The second type of change — using a different type of question to test the same ability — is feasible if another question type exists and if scoring comparability can be determined. For example, OPM is now conducting research on the feasibility of using symbolic tests with deaf applicants to substitute for our logic-based tests of verbal reasoning (Colberg, 1985).

The interpretive guidance to the EEOC's Title I regulations describes some rather bold substitutions of methods for measuring the same KSAs, as the following excerpt shows:

Where it is not possible to test in an alternative format, the employer may be required, as a reasonable accommodation, to evaluate the skill to be tested in another manner (e.g., through an interview, or through education, license, or work experience requirements) (EEOC, 1991, p. 35750).

This excerpt does not reflect a concern for score comparability. In fact, it is difficult to see how this approach could be used if applicants needed to be rank-ordered.

Changing or deleting a KSA would be justified only if there was no appropriate way to test the intended KSA and if there was reason to believe that it would not be required on the job by the disabled person. At the Office of Personnel Management, the practice is to sometimes delete test parts that are known to have the effect of screening out persons with certain disabilities because in large-scale, broad-band testing programs such as these one cannot be certain that there will not be some job that the person can fill. For example, speeded tests are deleted from the test battery for clerical jobs when visually or physically impaired persons apply. Their scores on the other test in the battery are prorated so that they can be put on the regular list of eligibles.

The interpretive guidance for EEOC's Title I regulations once again supports this type of change, as this excerpt indicates:

> ... an employer could require that an applicant complete a test within established time frames if speed were one of the skills for which the applicant was being tested. However, the results of such a test could not be used to exclude an individual with a disability unless the skill was necessary to perform an essential function of the position and no reasonable accommodation was available to enable the individual to perform that function, or the necessary accommodation would impose an undue hardship. (EEOC, 1991, p. 35750)

This interpretive guidance applies best to smaller-scale testing programs, in which reasonable accommodation can be considered for the position to be filled and for the testing instrument at the same time. Such programs in the context of state governments are described in Daley, Dollard, Kraft, Nester, and Schneider (1988).

Accommodation for Specific Disabilities

It is not possible to give readers of this book extensive background information on all the aspects of disabilities that might have an impact on employment testing. For a discussion of this topic, readers are advised to consult works by Bolton (1976), Levine (1960, 1974), Ziezula (1982), Scholl and Schnur (1976), Nester (1984), Van Rijn (1976), White (1978), and Willingham et al. (1988). Nevertheless, a brief listing of the types of testing accommodations that are appropriate for test-takers with different disabilities will be provided.

For test-takers with visual impairments, tests must be presented in appropriate media, such as braille, large print, and audiotape. Time limits must be extended for all these media, and speed tests are inappropriate. Within the context of changing test materials into different media, certain types of test material may be problematic, as noted earlier.

For test-takers who have physical impairments that affect use of the hands, the principal test accommodation is the adjustment of test time limits and the avoidance of speed tests.

Among hearing-impaired test-takers, only those who are deaf need extensive testing accommodations. For the majority of prelingually deaf persons who lost their hearing before acquiring speech, verbal tests are not good measures of any ability. Deaf persons, unlike the hearing, have low or no correlation between verbal and nonverbal test scores (Stunkel, 1957; Nester & Sapinkopf, 1982). It is as though verbal tests prevent deaf persons from showing their ability in any other field. As a result, verbal tests cannot be used with most deaf test-takers to test anything except verbal ability. In addition, test instructions should be given very carefully, with the use of sign language or demonstration, and time limits should be explained clearly. Extra time should be allowed on power tests that include verbal material.

Individuals with specific learning disabilities now constitute the largest group that requires testing accommodations. The specific tasks affected by learning disabilities vary widely, so it is impossible to generalize about testing accommodations. (Willingham et al., 1988, present an excellent discussion of the problems in characterizing the learning disabled group.) At OPM, we handle accommodations on a case-by-case basis for applicants with specific learning disabilities. The most frequently used accommodations are the allowance of additional time for power tests and deletion of some speed tests in areas of specific weakness.

Role of Rehabilitation Psychologists

It should come as no surprise to rehabilitation psychologists to learn that standard texts on educational and psychological testing have virtually no reference to testing persons with disabilities. This fact serves to illustrate that knowledge of this area is outside the mainstream of psychometrics. Perhaps in recognition of this problem, the Standards for Educational and Psychological Testing (AERA et al., 1985) specifically included a standard that requires expertise on the part of people who modify tests for handicapped persons. Clearly, rehabilitation psychologists can play a role in closing the "expertise gap" by sharing their specialized knowledge with testing organizations.

A second contribution is advocacy, in order to counter the resistance that ADA requirements for reasonable accommodation are bound to provoke. I see this advocacy as being dispassionate and firmly grounded on the technical knowledge held by rehabilitation psychologists that the capabilities of people with disabilities will make significant contributions in the workplace.

Acknowledgments

The opinions expressed in this chapter are the author's and do not necessarily represent the official policy of the U.S. Office of Personnel Management.

References

American Educational Research Association, American Psychological Association, & National Council on Measurement in Education (1985). *Standards for educational and psychological testing.* Washington, DC: American Psychological Association.

Bolton, B. (Ed.). (1976). *Handbook of measurement and evaluation in rehabilitation.* Baltimore: University Park Press.

Colberg, M. (1985). Logic-based measurement of verbal reasoning: A key to increased validity and economy. *Personnel Psychology, 38,* 347–359.

Daley, L., Dollard, M., Kraft, J. D., Nester, M. A., & Schneider, R. (1988). *Employment testing of persons with disabling conditions. Personnel Assessment Monograph, Vol. 1, No. 4.* Alexandria, VA: International Personnel Management Association Assessment Council.

Droege, R. C., & Mugaas, H. D. (1976). The USES testing program. In B. Bolton (Ed.), *Handbook of measurement and evaluation in rehabilitation* (pp. 187–206). Baltimore: University Park Press.

Equal Employment Opportunity Commission (1991). *Equal employment opportunity for individuals with disabilities.* Federal Register, 56, 35725–35753.

Heaton, S. M., Nelson, A. V., & Nester, M. A. (1980). *Guide for administering examinations to handicapped individuals for employment purposes* (PRR 80-16). Washington, DC: U.S. Office of Personnel Management.

Levine, E. S. (1960). *The psychology of deafness: Techniques of appraisal for rehabilitation.* New York: Columbia University Press.

Levine, E. S. (1974). *Psychological tests and practices with the deaf. A survey of the state of the art.* The Volta Review, 76, 298–319.

Nester, M. A. (1984). *Employment testing for handicapped people.* Public Personnel Management, 13, 417–434.

Nester, M. A., & Sapinkopf, R. C. (1982). *A Federal employment test modified for deaf applicants* (OPRD 82-7). Washington, DC: U.S. Office of Personnel Management.

Nunnally, J. (1978). *Psychometric theory (2nd. ed.)*. New York: McGraw-Hill.

Sapinkopf, R. C. (1978). *Statistical characteristics of the written test for the Professional and Administrative Career Examination (PACE) for visually handicapped applicants* (TM 78-1). Washington, DC: U.S. Civil Service Commission.

Scholl, C., & Schnur, R. (1976). *Measures of psychological, vocational, and educational functioning in the blind and visually handicapped*. New York: American Foundation for the Blind.

Sherman, S. W., & Anderson, N. M. (Eds.). (1982). *Ability testing of handicapped people: Dilemma for government, science, and the public*. Washington, DC: National Academy Press.

Shultz, M., & Boynton, M. (1958). *Typing tests: Visual copy vs. recordings*. Public Personnel Review, 19, 24-27.

Stunkel, E. R. (1957). The performance of deaf and hearing college students on verbal and non-verbal intelligence tests. *American Annals of the Deaf*, 102, 342-355.

U.S. Civil Service Commission (1956). *Tests for blind competitors for trades and industrial jobs in the Federal Civil Service*. Washington, DC: Author.

U.S. Department of Health, Education, and Welfare (1977). *Nondiscrimination on the basis of handicap*. Federal Register, 42, 22677-22694.

U.S. Department of Labor, Manpower Administration (1970). *Manual for the USTES General Aptitude Test Battery, Section III: Development*. Washington, DC: U.S. Government Printing Office.

van Rijn, P. (1976). *Testing the handicapped for employment purposes: Some adaptations for persons with dyslexia* (PS 76-4). Washington, DC: Personnel Research and Development Center, U.S. Civil Service Commission.

White, K. O. (1978). *Testing the handicapped for employment purposes: Adaptations for persons with motor handicaps* (PS 78-4). Washington, DC: Personnel Research and Development Center, U.S. Civil Service Commission.

Willingham, W. W., Ragosta, M., Bennett, R. E., Braun, H., Rock, D. A., &

Powers, D. E. (1988). *Testing handicapped people*. Boston: Allyn and Bacon, Inc.

Ziezula, F. R. (Ed.). (1982). *Assessment of hearing-impaired people: A guide for selecting psychological, educational, and vocational tests*. Washington, DC: Gallaudet College Press.

· 4 ·

The ADA and the Hiring Process in Organizations

Richard Klimoski and Susan N. Palmer

Overview

"Having a stable and fulfilling job is a basic component of the American Dream. Every one of us would like to have a job that is enjoyable and stimulating and that provides us with sufficient income to meet our needs. People with disabilities are no different" (Feldblum, 1991, p. 82).

Our chapter is being written with this quote in mind. An over-arching goal of the Americans with Disabilities Act (ADA) is to help create a society where individuals with disabilities can expect to be employed to their fullest potential. However, we feel that to do this, it is imperative that consultants and human resource professionals find ways to insure that the best interests of both job applicants with disabilities and the best interests of hiring organizations are met in the design and execution of organizational recruitment and assessment practices. This is frequently a challenge. Such consultants and professionals have the skills and technical expertise necessary to help organizations meet this challenge. They are certainly well-positioned to have some type of impact. With this chapter we are trying to ensure that this impact will be positive.

Objectives for this Chapter

More specifically, here are some of our objectives in writing this chapter:

a) We seek to motivate compliance with the provisions of the ADA by those professionals charged with staffing responsibilities in their organizations. In fact, we hope to show that attention to the intent and not just the letter of the law will prove to be in the best interests of the organization. In this regard, we take what might be characterized as an optimistic and positive view of the impact of the Act, as it has the potential of promoting the availability of a new pool of potentially suitable applicants, those that have both the ability and motivation to be productive (Rynes & Barber, 1990).

b) Many employers utilize psychological testing and assessment as part of the hiring process. Thus it is necessary to understand how such procedures will need to be altered to provide reasonable accommodations and what issues and potential problems might arise with such alterations. Toward this end, we summarize the logic of scientific personnel selection. For many readers this will serve as a review. For all readers it provides a reminder of the working assumptions that staffing specialists usually hold. We also will use a generalized case to illustrate when, where, and how selection systems in large decentralized companies (where accommodation policies will be most difficult to carry out) might be modified to accommodate individuals with a disability, while at the same time remaining true to scientific and professional standards.

c) We will stress collaboration and cooperation as key to the successful implementation of requests for accommodation under the ADA. Both the applicant and the professionals representing the organization have a role to play. Thus, Chapter 4 will outline when and in what ways this collaboration might occur, using our case example.

d) Finally, we wish to promote the notion of, and need for, the continuous adaptation of personnel selection programs to changing conditions. In this regard, we emphasize the need for corporate learning and continuous improvement in the process of providing for those who seek accommodation under the ADA. While we can offer some insights on implementation based on our understanding of the Act, and on the impact of the Rehabilitation Act of 1973, corporate experience to date is limited. Thus we will advocate data gathering and feedback systems to ensure that future papers on personnel selection systems in industry, under the ADA, will be better grounded in research and practice (see Campbell, 1969).

The Nature of Personnel Selection

Scientifically based personnel selection principles have been available for over 70 years. By the second decade in this century in the United States, industrial/organizational psychologists such as Scott (1911) and Munsterberg (1913) were working with a variety of companies to improve the accuracy of personnel selection. Scott was later to use his expertise to advise the U.S. Military during the First World War on the processing and screening of over 1,700,000 men. In the years since, a great deal of empirical research has been carried out on approaches to personnel selection. Moreover, a great deal of practical wisdom has also accumulated (Katzell & Austin, 1992). Thus by the 1980s, Schmidt, Hunter, and their colleagues (Schmidt & Hunter, 1981; Schmidt, Hunter, McKenzie & Muldrow, 1979; Schmidt, Hunter & Pearlman, 1982) were able to point out both the real (scientifically established) and financial and practical benefits of systematic and professionally based personnel selection practices (Schmitt & Borman, 1993). It would be prudent for anyone who is interested in shaping approaches to staffing in the context of implementing the ADA to revisit the nature of these long-established scientifically based principles and practices in order to build on them.

The Logic of Personnel Selection

The logic of personnel selection is based on the very nature of modern complex organizations and on the practice of a division of labor and job responsibilities (specialization) that has evolved over the years. It is also related to the realities and logistics of recruiting and hiring people.

Whether the job involved is that of a sales person or a computer operator there will be a set of worker requirements. These are the knowledge, the skills, the abilities, the needs, the motives and the personality dispositions needed to perform. To put it another way, these are the important job requirements and personal attributes of the people who are likely to be successful on the job.

The preferred starting point for identifying worker requirements is to conduct a job analysis. There are a variety of ways to do this (Gael, 1987; Levine, 1983) but often it involves a selection specialist who will observe workers performing the job in question, examine the context of the job, conduct interviews with workers and their bosses, and occasionally make use of a specially constructed questionnaire to be completed by incumbents. A good job analysis is systematic, makes use of a variety of techniques, and is carried out by a qualified individual. The objective is to get as complete and accurate a picture of the job as possible. Without one, efforts at recruiting and selecting people will be seriously flawed and may place the organization in legal jeopardy in the event of challenges to the selection system.

Although a wide variety of worker requirements have been identified, for purposes of this chapter, it will be convenient to cluster them into two types. Selection specialists often distinguish between what might be called "can do" requirements vs. "will do" requirements (Porter, Lawler, and Hackman, 1975). As implied, the "can do" requirements are those knowledge, skills, and abilities which determine whether or not a person is likely to be ABLE to do the job assuming that he or she put out some work effort. This can be thought of as the capacity to perform. In fact, "can do" requirements limit the potential of an individual for effective job performance in important ways (Blumberg & Pringle, 1983).

In contrast, other characteristics might be important for success because they imply how motivated a person is likely to be if placed on the job. Extensive research has established that interests, values, or needs must be met or fulfilled on the job for people to be motivated (e.g., Wanous, 1980). Thus "will do" requirements describe the potential of the job to satisfy certain needs, or alternatively, the needs of certain types of individuals.

Any given job will typically have both types of requirements. To be effective, a newly hired person will usually have to meet both sets. To put it another way, if a person can't do the job (for lack of ability) it is unlikely that high levels of motivation alone will be sufficient. However, even if the individual does have the ability to do the job, he or she may not demonstrate the motivation or the inclination to do the job once placed there. In fact, there is ample evidence that fully capable individuals hired into a job which fails to meet their needs are very likely to quit in short order (Wanous, 1980). Most jobs will demand a mixture of "can do" and "will do" factors in order to be successful.

Measuring Worker Requirements

Over the years, selection specialists have developed different ways of measuring or estimating the extent that applicants meet or exceed job requirements. Some of these approaches are more appropriate for assessing a candidate's capabilities; others, for assessing his/her needs and values. Figure 4.1 lists some examples.

Often, a given selection technique is used to get at a wide range of applicant qualifications. That is, it attempts to get at both the ability and motivational requirements of the job. Thus, in most organizations, a selection interview is involved in the screening of candidates in the belief that, in fact, in a carefully designed and conducted interview, a wide range of qualities may be assessed (Campion, Pursell, & Brown, 1988). In addition, an organization might use a test battery made up of different kinds of tests (ability and personality) to assess critical factors.

Establishing the Usefulness of a Selection Device

Prior to actually implementing a particular approach to selection or adopting a specific device, it is important to establish that it will, in fact, be useful. This is the essence of personnel research in most organizations. Selection specialists will do this by comparing what is known about the device to

Type of Information Obtained	Type of Measure
Maximum Performance "Can Do"	Cognitive Tests
	Aptitude Tests
	Work Sample Tests
	Physical Ability Tests
	Assessment Centers
Typical Behavior "Will Do"	Biographical Data
	Personality Measures
Both	Employment Interview
	Reference Checks

Figure 4.1 Measuring worker requirements.
(From Schmitt and Klimoski, 1991.)

a set of standards. Several of these standards will be only briefly men tioned as they are detailed elsewhere (Schmitt & Klimoski, 1991). Others will be given greater attention because they are especially relevant to the implementation of the ADA.

Reliability

The essence of reliability is consistency of measurement. More technically, reliability refers to the extent that data or information obtained with a partic-ular measurement tool or selection device is free from errors (Schmitt & Klimoski, 1991). There are a variety of ways to estimate reliability. Depending on the purpose(s) of the measure or assessment device, they will be differentially relevant. In staffing, repeated measures reliability (for tests) and inter-judge reliability (for interviews) are important. It is not uncommon to get multiple estimates of reliability in the development of selection devices.

Validity

While we make some distinctions below regarding content, construct, and criterion-related validity, we do so to facilitate presentation. Current think-ing about validity in assessment contexts plays down these distinctions and instead emphasizes the quality and strength of inferences that are made based on evidence (Kane, 1992; Landy, 1986; Schmitt & Landy, 1992). Thus it is incorrect to emphasize the validity of a test without clear refer-ence to the context of the decisions to be made (e.g., does the test measure a constant?; are we assessing current abilities?; do we have an accurate esti-mate of a person's potential for future assignments?).

Content Validity

Whenever we want to be certain that a selection device is measuring all of the important worker requirements, we raise the issue of content validity. More technically, content validity refers to the degree to which the responses required by the test or measure are a representative sample of the whole domain of performance-related behaviors or types of knowledge that are important to the job. In the case of personnel selection, it usually means that our criterion measure captures the essential features of effective job performances and that we really are measuring the key qualifications needed for this performance. That is to say, we want content validity for both our selection devices and any measures of effectiveness that we might use in developing such devices.

Construct Validity

In many instances we assume that a selection device or measure is getting at some underlying theme, or, more technically, some construct. Thus, a cognitive ability test is presumed to be measuring aspects of intellectual functioning; an honesty test, honesty, etc. Alternatively, an interview may or may not be used to assess the candidate's level or score relative to the notion (construct) of the good employee. It would depend on what questions were asked and the kinds of inferences that are made. For example, the answer to a question whereby the applicant is asked to describe his/her experiences working under deadlines or time pressure may be noted as merely descriptive of past work experience or may be used to infer how much "resilience" (a construct) the applicant possesses.

Criterion-Related Validity

This refers to empirical evidence obtained with an assessment device which are related to some important set of behaviors or some level of functioning. In personnel selection, persuasive evidence of criterion-related validity would be to show that scores on a selection device are in fact related to aspects of job performance.

Utility

Most selection devices are intended to be used for personnel decision making. The assumption is that by using the device, the organization is improving the likelihood that those people who are recommended for hire will be better than those who are rejected. But we expect even more when we introduce a new device. We assume that among those who are selected with a new device we will find a larger proportion of individuals who will be viewed as successful (on the job), over what we are currently getting by using traditional methods. Utility, usually expressed in cost-benefit or dollar terms, refers to the extent that a measure does indeed fulfill this promise (Cascio, 1982; Fitz-Enz, 1984; Spencer, 1986). We usually establish utility by demonstrating that we are making fewer selection errors by using the selection device than we would by not using it. An important point here is that specialists have traditionally thought of worker qualifications in terms of probabilities and/or degrees of success. Only recently has it become common to find organizations making reference to the dichotomy of qualified/unqualified applicant.

The latter implies that in personnel work there will always be some chance of making a decision error. No known selection system exists where this is not the case. In utility analysis, the particular kinds of errors (e.g., "false positives") made when using a selection device are examined. When selecting personnel, mistakes can indeed be costly. For example, a recent survey of U.S. personnel officers of large private companies revealed that on average it costs over $18,000 to dismiss an employee (Fowler, 1990). It is thus possible to estimate the money saved by using a particular device. However, utility would not only involve this figure (the benefits of avoiding mistakes), but an analysis of the actual expenses incurred in developing the measure and the recurring expenses associated with its use.

To be complete, estimating utility would also require us to consider the relative costs and benefits of alternatives. For instance, there might be some other very inexpensive approach to selection that works almost as well.

Freedom From Bias

In the United States today it is public policy to ensure equal employment opportunities for all people regardless of religion, sex, nationality, disability, race, or ethnic background. It is also against the law to unfairly discriminate in employment practices. Thus, the impact of a selection device must be scrutinized to see if there are disproportionate numbers of individuals in these protected classes who are adversely impacted. (See Reilly & Chao, 1982, or Arvey & Faley, 1988, for a good review of the issues involved in this area.) When it comes to indexing fair treatment of a person with a disability, under the ADA, it remains to be seen just what kind of evidence will be found acceptable to all the parties involved (applicant/ incumbent, hiring organization, courts, etc). More will be said about this later.

Acceptance

Most of the standards listed so far have a strong technical component. In the case of acceptance, we are simply stating that a selection device must be perceived as appropriate and fair to the people involved. In technical terms, this is face validity—that the tool being used has items that are appropriate to the target group and are perceived as being relevant. For example, a test of sales aptitude for selection of sales representatives has items that are sales-related rather than, say, engineering-related. Such groups would include job applicants, those people ultimately hired, current workers and managers of the organization, as well as the human resource professionals involved (recruiters, trainers). User acceptance is very often a function of the care taken in the development of the device. It is affected by the kind of evidence (quality and quantity) that exists for its validity. But perceptions of fairness and appropriateness will also be related to how, and by what means, the selection tool was implemented or put into practice. Unilateral imposition of new hiring standards and/or the initial widespread use of particular screening programs (e.g., drug testing via urine samples) is likely to produce low acceptance, irrespective of what validity or utility evidence exists. In the same vein, some modifications or forms of accommodation in selection screening procedures may also create negative reactions if not introduced in an appropriate manner (see Gilliland, in press).

Robustness

This concept reflects the extent to which an assessment or selection device can be administered using a variety of forms or modalities and still retain its ability to produce correct inferences regarding the suitability of a candidate for a position (Brinberg & McGrath, 1985). A device that is robust would allow more flexibility in the way that it is applied or taken. Generally speaking, it would seem desirable to identify or develop measures that are relatively unaffected by changes in administration as would occur in response to a request for accommodation. For example, a numerical aptitude test might be developed that allows for the same valid inference of an applicant's capabilities in this area whether it is administered in a traditional printed version, a Braille edition, orally, or on a customized, portable computer (which might be used by individuals with limited use of their hands). We would still recommend however, that despite a high degree of robustness, a paper-and-pencil instrument should still be revalidated if it is converted to a radically different format, whenever it is technically possible (see Tenopyr et. al., 1993).

This set of standards is most often applied to paper-and-pencil tests or inventories. However, they should be used in discussing the usefulness of any potential personnel selection device or program. That is to say, we would expect that an interview used as a decision aid for selection would yield information that exhibits reliability, validity, utility, etc.

To locate or develop selection/assessment procedures that comply with the above standards will take a great deal of time, money and effort. Thus, when an organization has a set of procedures that meets its needs, there is a great deal of pressure to protect it from compromise. Practically speaking, this implies that the managers responsible for selection programs will be motivated toward consistency in application. To put it differently, such individuals would normally be reluctant to make changes in practice unless there are compelling reasons to do so (i.e., a legitimate request for accommodation).

Key Provisions of the ADA

Title I of the ADA, the employment title of the Act, focuses on the employment of individuals with disabilities. Employers cannot discriminate against individuals with disabilities in regard to employment practices, or the terms, conditions, and privileges of employment (Americans with Disabilities Act, I-4) including:

• application	• disciplinary actions
• termination	• testing
• training	• compensation
• hiring	• promotion
• leave	• assignments
• medical exams	• layoff/recall
• evaluation	• benefits

ADA requirements for nondiscrimination in employment became effective for employers with 25 or more employees on July 26, 1992, and will extend to employers with 15 to 24 employees on July 26, 1994.

The ADA does not guarantee equal outcomes, establish quotas, or require preferences favoring individuals with disabilities over individuals without disabilities. Rather, the ADA is intended to ensure access to equal employment opportunities based on merit. The ADA is designed to "level the playing field" by removing the barriers that prevent qualified individuals with disabilities from having access to the same employment opportunities that are available to qualified individuals without disabilities.

Overview of Legal Requirements

In this section we will give an overview of the employment title of the ADA with particular emphasis on the sections that cover the hiring process. This is not intended to be a comprehensive review of the Act or to repeat what appears in other articles in this volume. Rather, this overview is offered as a reference for some of the specific employment issues covered in this article.

The ADA prohibits employment discrimination against "qualified individuals with disabilities" (Americans with Disabilities Act, 1992, I-2). The ADA definition of an "individual with a disability" is an individual who:

- has a physical or mental impairment that substantially limits one or more of his/her life activities;

- has a record of such an impairment; or

- is regarded as having such an impairment.

Thus, the ADA definition of "disability" is broad and comprehensive. The Act lists many but not all conditions that make up physical or mental impairments given the variety of possible impairments (Americans with Disabilities Act, 1992, II-2). In the ADA, a physical impairment is defined as: "any physiological disorder or condition, cosmetic disfigurement, or anatomical loss affecting one or more of the following body systems: neurological, musculoskeletal, special sense organs, respiratory (including speech organs), cardiovascular, reproductive, digestive, genito-urinary, hemic and lymphatic, skin, and endocrine." The Act defines a mental impairment as: "any mental or psychological disorder such as mental retardation, organic brain syndrome, emotional or mental illness, and specific learning disabilities."

While current drug users are not protected as individuals with disabilities, former drug users and individuals undergoing rehabilitation are protected as long as they are not currently using illegal drugs (see Segal, 1992; Jones, Chapter 8). Conditions which are not considered impairments include environmental, cultural, or economic disadvantages (e.g., poverty, lack of education, prison record). Personality traits (e.g., poor judgment, quick temper) are not by themselves impairments but may be if they are symptoms of a physical or mental disorder. In addition, physical characteristics such as eye or hair color, lefthandedness, or height or weight within a normal range are not considered impairments. Having a physical or mental impairment is only part of the first definition. An impairment must also substantially limit one or more major life activities (Americans with Disabilities Act, 1992, II-3 to II-6) such as walking, speaking, breathing, performing manual tasks, seeing, hearing, learning, caring for oneself, or working. Factors to consider in determining whether or not an impairment substantially limits a major life activity include:

- its nature and severity;

- how long it will last or is expected to last;

- its permanent or long-term impact, or expected impact.

Temporary or minor impairments (e.g., broken bones, influenza) that do not last for a long time, or have little impact, are not generally considered disabilities protected by the ADA.

In discussing the major life activity of working (Americans with Disabilities Act, 1992, II-6 to II-7), the term "substantially limited," means that an individual is significantly restricted in the ability to perform an entire class of jobs, or a broad range of jobs in various classes, as compared to the average person with similar training, skills, and abilities. If the individual is unable to perform a single particular job, the individual is not necessarily "substantially limited," with respect to the major life activity of working. Factors to help determine if an individual is substantially limited in working include:

- the type of job from which the individual has been disqualified because of the impairment;

- the geographical area in which the person may reasonably expect to find a job;

- the number and types of jobs using similar training, knowledge, skill, or abilities from which the individual is disqualified within the geographical area; and/or

- the number and types of other jobs in the area that do not involve similar training, knowledge, skills, or abilities from which the individual also is disqualified because of the impairment.

The second definition of disability covers individuals who have a history of an impairment or who have been diagnosed, either correctly or incorrectly as having an impairment, whether or not they currently are substantially limited in a major life activity (Americans with Disabilities Act, 1992, II-8). The ADA thus protects individuals who have recovered from a physical or mental impairment (e.g., cancer, heart disease, mental illness) as well as individuals who may have been misclassified as having an impairment (e.g., mental retardation, learning disability).

The third definition of a disability covers an individual who either does not have an impairment (e.g., rumor that an individual is HIV positive) or does not have an impairment that substantially limits major life activities (e.g., controlled high blood pressure) but is regarded as having such an impairment. This definition is specifically intended to protect individuals from a range of discriminatory actions based on "myths, fears and stereotypes" (Americans with Disabilities Act, 1992, II-10).

In addition to protecting individuals with disabilities, the ADA also protects individuals who have a relationship (e.g., spouse) or association (e.g., volunteer work) with individuals with disabilities. For example, if an applicant without a disability discloses in an interview that he/she has a spouse who is disabled, the employer cannot decline to hire the applicant because the employer is concerned about the applicant's future work attendance or the possible impact on the company's health benefits plan. This broad and comprehensive definition of a "disability" establishes a threshold for ADA protection, and individuals who do not fall within one of the above categories will not be covered under the ADA (Feldblum, 1991). The Act also requires that the person be a "qualified individual with a disability." A "qualified individual with a disability" is:

"an individual with a disability who meets the skill, experience, education, and other job-related requirements of a position held or desired, and who, with or without reasonable accommodation, can perform the essential functions of the job." (Americans with Disabilities Act, 1992, I-3)

Thus, an employer is not required to hire or retain an individual who is not qualified to perform the job. In determining whether an individual is qualified under the ADA, the employer needs to first determine if the individual meets the necessary prerequisites for the job (Americans with Disabilities Act, 1992, II-11 to II-12) such as:

- education   • work

- experience   • licenses

- training   • other job-related experience.

This step is sometimes referred to as determining if an individual with a disability is "otherwise qualified." For example, if an employer is hiring a lawyer for its legal department, does the individual have a law degree and is he/she licensed to practice law in the state? An individual with a disability is otherwise qualified if he/she has the credentials for the job, but due to a disability may need reasonable accommodation to perform the job's essential functions (Americans with Disabilities Act, 1992, Appendix B, B-41).

If the individual with a disability meets the necessary job prerequisites, then the employer needs to determine if the individual can perform the essential functions of the job, with or without reasonable accommodation (Americans with Disabilities Act, 1992, II-12). This is a key aspect of nondiscrimination under the ADA in order to prevent discrimination against individuals with disabilities who can perform the essential job functions but may not be able to perform functions that are marginal or tangential to the job.

The ADA lists several reasons why a function could be considered essential to a job (Americans with Disabilities Act, 1992, II-13 to II-14). These include:

- the position exists to perform the function;

- there are a limited number of other employees available to perform the function, or among whom the function can be distributed; or

- a function is highly specialized, and the person in the position is hired for special expertise or ability to perform it.

The ADA also lists what type of evidence can be used in determining whether a function is essential (Americans with Disabilities Act, 1992, II-14 to II-17). Evidence to be considered include:

- the employer's judgment (especially as backed up by a job analysis);

- a written job description prepared before advertising or interviewing applicants for a job;

- the amount of time spent performing the function;

- the consequences of not requiring a person in this job to perform a function;

- the terms of a collective bargaining agreement;

- work experience of people who have performed a job in the past and work experience of people who currently perform similar jobs; and

- other relevant factors.

While an employer can establish what a job is and what functions are required to perform this job, the ADA requires that an individual with a disability be considered relative to the job's essential functions. An employer must also make the determination of whether an individual is qualified or not, based on the individual's qualifications at the time of the employment decision in question, not on speculation that the individual may become unable to do so in the future (Americans with Disabilities Act, 1992, Appendix B, B-18).

Many individuals with disabilities are able to perform the essential functions of jobs. However, if an individual with a disability who is otherwise qualified for the job cannot perform one or more of the essential job functions due to his/her disability, it is the employer's responsibility to determine if that individual is qualified for the job when a modification or adjustment to the job would enable the individual to perform the essential functions. This key nondiscrimination requirement of the ADA is known as "reasonable accommodation" (Americans with Disabilities Act, 1992, III-1 to III-3).

"Reasonable accommodation" is a modification or adjustment to the job, the work environment, or the way things are customarily done that enables an individual with a disability to enjoy equal employment opportunities (Americans with Disabilities Act, 1992, III-2). The ADA requires reasonable accommodation in three aspects of employment:

- to ensure equal opportunity in the application process;

- to enable a qualified individual with a disability to perform the essential functions of a job; and

- to enable an employee with a disability to enjoy equal benefits and privileges of employment.

For purposes of this chapter, we will highlight reasonable accommodation that would enable a qualified applicant with a disability to have an equal opportunity in the hiring process.

Finally, the ADA expressly prohibits employers from using qualification standards, employment tests, or other selection criteria that screen out or tend to screen out an individual with a disability unless the selection criteria are clearly job-related and can be justified by business necessity (Americans with Disabilities Act, 1992, IV-1). The ADA requirements apply to all selection standards and procedures including:

- education and work experience requirements;

- physical and mental requirements;

- safety requirements;

- paper-and-pencil tests;

- physical or psychological tests;

- interview questions; and

- rating systems.

Selection criteria that exclude or tend to exclude individuals with disabilities but do not relate to an essential function of a job would not be viewed as being consistent with business necessity. Those that are related to essential functions would be. However, even the latter may not be used to exclude applicants with disabilities if these individuals could satisfy the criteria by using reasonable accommodation (Americans with Disabilities Act, 1992, Appendix B, B-47).

Preparing for Equal Opportunity in the Hiring Process

Given the above legal requirements, consultants and human resource professionals should help an employer carefully review all of its policies and procedures used in recruiting and selecting employees to ensure that individuals with disabilities have equal opportunities to participate in the hiring process and to be considered for a job. While the ADA does not require employers to recruit and select specifically individuals with disabilities (e.g., there is no affirmative action objective), recruitment and selection activities that cannot be shown to be job-related or that have the effect of screening out applicants with disabilities may violate the ADA (Americans with Disabilities Act, 1992, V-3). In this section we will cover the hiring activities of recruitment, pre-employment inquiries (e.g., application forms, reference checks), interviewing, employment testing, and medical examinations, as most employers use one or more of these activities when recruiting and selecting employees for job openings. The information provided will assist consultants and human resource professionals working with employers to identify and revise any practice that may be inconsistent with the ADA's nondiscrimination requirements.

Recruitment

Because individuals with disabilities represent a large, underutilized applicant pool, in their desire to hire and retain a qualified workforce, many employers have expanded their outreach sources to include qualified individuals with disabilities. There are many sources for locating individuals (Americans with Disabilities Act, 1992, V-4) with disabilities who are qualified for job openings including:

- state and local vocational rehabilitation agencies;

- occupational therapists;

- local centers for independent living;

- organizations representing people who have specific disabilities; and

- coordinators of student service programs at colleges and universities.

For a comprehensive list of other recruitment sources see the Resource Directory Index in the ADA Technical Assistance Manual.

Employers are also advised to review their job announcements, advertisements, and other recruitment materials for wording that will "screen in" rather than "screen out" qualified individuals with disabilities. For example, a job announcement may indicate that "oral communication skills" are needed for the job when the incumbent could, in fact, communicate effectively using non-oral methods such as a written memo or electronic mail message. Finally, employers may also want to include in their job announcements, advertisements, and recruitment materials, a statement that they do not discriminate on the basis of disability or other legally prohibited bases.

Figures 4.2(a) and (b) illustrate an "old" and "new" job description for a customer service representative. The "new" description has been prepared to be responsive to the Act's call for a focus on essential functions. It is offered in contrast to the more traditional job description to emphasize the more specific wording that is recommended under the ADA. A rule of thumb used to guide the creation of the new description was to consider the applicant's point of view. In our view, a good job description is one that informs the applicant of the nature of the work to be performed to a level of detail or specificity that allows for what might be termed "informed choice." In this regard, it operates much like a "realistic job preview" (Wanous, 1980).

Job Responsibilities:

- Answer customer phone calls.
- Gather customer information.
- Resolve customer complaints.
- Write customers regarding status of inquiry or complaint.
- Document customer contacts.
- Operate a PC and/or CRT.

Required Knowledge, Skills, and Abilities:

- Knowledge of company's products and services.
- Oral communication skills.
- Written communication skills.
- Problem-solving skills.
- Interpersonal skills.
- Organizational skill
- Basic math skills.

**Figure 4.2(a) Original job description:
Customer service representative.**

Employers should check to see if information about job openings is accessible to individuals with different disabilities. For instance, job information could be available to individuals with mobility impairments in physically accessible sites; to individuals with hearing impairments through a Telecommunications Device for the Deaf (TDD) phone number; or to individuals with visual impairments through large print, audio cassette, or a telephone recording.

Many employers use employment agencies to assist them in recruiting, screening, and referring applicants. These agencies are "covered entities" under the ADA and must comply with all ADA requirements. Since the employer may also be liable if there is any violation of ADA requirements by the agency, an employer should inform the agency of the mutual obligation to comply with ADA requirements. The employer should consider informing the agency of the mutual obligation through a letter or a provision in the written contract, reviewing the agency's written materials for a nondiscrimination statement, and discussing the agency's procedures regarding pre-employment inquiries and reasonable accommodation.

Pre-Employment Inquiries

The ADA specifically prohibits an employer from making any pre-employment inquiries about a disability or about the nature or severity of a disability

Job Responsibilities:

- Provide timely, accurate, and complete customer account and product information to customers via telephone.

- Offer products and services to customers via telephone.

- Make telephone calls to customers to gather information that is missing or unclear on incoming applications or orders.

- Conduct required account research to resolve customer inquiries or complaints.

- Identify problems and determine appropriate actions to be taken to resolve customer inquiries or complaints.

- Respond in writing regarding status of customer inquiries or complaints.

- Compose written documentation of customer contacts for internal and external use.

- Perform data base input and report generation using a PC and/or CRT.

Required Knowledge, Skills, and Abilities:

- Knowledge of company's products, services, operations, and policies.

- Ability to receive and understand spoken information from others.

- Ability to orally communicate information to others.

- Ability to read and understand company policies and procedures.

- Ability to clearly and concisely communicate information in writing.

- Ability to apply company policies and procedures to a customer problem and develop a logical answer.

- Ability to interact effectively and courteously with customers, vendors, and other company employees, particularly irate customers.

- Ability to perform basic mathematical operations (e.g., add, subtract, multiply, divide, etc.).

- Ability to operate a PC and/or CRT terminal including typing and 10-key input.

- Ability to work independently with minimal supervision.

- Ability to organize, prioritize, and complete multiple concurrent tasks under tight time constraints in a high volume environment.

Figure 4.2 (b) Revised job description: Customer service representative.

(Americans with Disabilities Act, 1992, V-5). This prohibition specifically impacts the information that can and cannot be requested on application forms, in job interviews, or in background or reference checks that are used as part of the staffing process. This prohibition does not prevent an employer from obtaining information about the individual's ability to perform specific job functions including asking an individual with a disability to describe or demonstrate how he/she would perform these functions. This prohibition is designed to ensure that qualified individuals are not screened out because of their disabilities before their actual abilities to do a job can be evaluated.

Employers should review their job application forms to eliminate any questions that could be related to a disability such as:

- "Please list any conditions or diseases for which you have been treated in the past 3 years."

- "Have you ever been hospitalized? If so, for what condition?"

- "Is there any health-related reason you may not be able to perform the job for which you are applying?"

- "Have you ever been treated for drug addiction or alcoholism?"

- "Have you ever filed a workers' compensation claim?"

Before making a job offer, many employers request information about a job applicant from previous employers or other sources. Under the ADA (Americans with Disabilities Act, 1992, V-17),when making background and reference checks, employers may not ask about an applicant's disability, illness, or worker's compensation history. Instead, the employer is encouraged to focus on the job functions and tasks performed by the applicant, the quality and quantity of work performed, attendance record, or other job-related issues that do not directly relate to a disability.

Interviewing

An employer should also review its structured interview forms and/or train its interviewers on what may and may not be asked during an interview. The basic requirements about pre-employment inquiries are also applicable here. In general, emphasis should be placed on the applicant's ability to perform essential functions of the job, not on a disability (Americans with Disabilities Act, 1992, V-10 to V-14).

An interviewer may obtain information about an applicant's ability to perform essential job functions and, with certain limitations, about any need for accommodation. Some general interviewing guidelines include:

- An applicant may be asked to describe or demonstrate how

he/she will perform specific job functions if this is required of everyone applying for a job in this job category. For example, an interviewer may ask an applicant to describe or demonstrate how he/she would lift a 50 lb. box if this lifting requirement is required to do the job. However, an interviewer should avoid asking whether the applicant has back problems.

- If an applicant has a known disability that would appear to interfere with or prevent performance of a job-related function, he/she may be asked to describe or demonstrate how this function would be performed, even if other applicants do not have to do so. For example, an interviewer may ask an applicant with one arm to describe or demonstrate how he/she would file small index cards if this filing is required for the job even if other applicants are not asked this. However, the interviewer cannot ask how the applicant lost his/her arm.

- If an applicant has a known disability that would not interfere with or prevent performance of a job-related function, the employer can only ask the applicant to describe or demonstrate how he/she would perform the function if all applicants in the job category are required to do so. For example, an interviewer may not ask an applicant in a wheelchair to describe or demonstrate how he/she would answer customer phone calls at a console unless all applicants for the job would be asked to demonstrate this as well.

If there is a requirement that individuals in an interview setting demonstrate how they would perform a job-related function (as in a work sample exercise), the employer may need to provide a reasonable accommodation to enable an applicant with a disability to perform to his/her potential.

Employment Testing

Many employers use employment tests to assist them in choosing among job applicants or employees when making decisions regarding qualifications for hiring, transfer, promotion, and other employment decisions. Depending upon the job requirements, these tests may be designed to evaluate job knowledge, skills and abilities, or other characteristics that are necessary for successful job performance.

As mentioned earlier, employment tests have been found to be among the best types of selection devices (see also Schmitt, Gooding, Noe and Kirsch, 1984). Thus, it is no coincidence that many organizations rely on them to identify the best candidates for employment. While the ADA does not prohibit the use of employment tests in the hiring process, the ADA does have two major requirements for employers who use tests to determine job qualifications (Americans with Disabilities Act, 1992, V-17 to V-21).

First, a test that screens out or tends to screen out an individual with a disability on the basis of the disability must be job-related and consistent with business necessity. This requirement applies to all types of employment tests including job knowledge, skills, aptitude, physical agility, work samples, etc.

Second, tests must reflect the skills and aptitudes of an individual rather than impaired sensory (including the abilities to hear, see, and process information), manual, or speaking skills, unless those are job-related skills the test is designed to measure. The purpose of this requirement is to ensure that the tests accurately reflect an individual's skills and aptitudes rather than the individual's impaired skills, and does not therefore exclude them from jobs that they can do because the disability prevents them from taking a test, or because it negatively influences the test results.

The notion of reasonable accommodation in the administration of employment tests is similar in logic to what we have emphasized in the other sections. However, the execution of this logic is far more problematic, as there are few recommendations or general rules that can be offered on how best to do this. Of all the aspects associated with the hiring process (e.g., recruiting, interviewing), we feel that accommodation in employment testing has the potential to be the most contentious. Therefore, in light of the importance of testing to the hiring process in large organizations and the complexity of the issues involved, much of the material in the remainder of this chapter will relate to, or at least touch upon, this issue.

Medical Examinations

Many employers include medical examinations or histories as part of their hiring process. This falls into the area of pre-employment inquiries (see above section) under the ADA and is specifically prohibited prior to making a conditional job offer (Americans with Disabilities Act, 1992, IV-1). Employers will need to adjust the timing of medical examinations as the ADA only permits post-offer, pre-employment medical examinations. Under the ADA, tests for illegal use of drugs are not considered medical examinations (Americans with Disabilities Act, 1992, B-64). In addition, an employer may only require a post-offer, pre-employment medical examination if:

- the employer has made an offer of employment that is conditioned on the results of the examination;

- all entering employees are subject to the same examination; and

- the results of the examination are treated as confidential medical records.

At the time of this writing, there is considerable discussion as to whether or not personality-oriented employment tests are medical examinations as defined by the ADA. The resolution of this issue is very important because if employment tests are viewed as medical examinations, then these tests could only be made after a conditional offer of employment is made. In our opinion, an employment test should not be considered a medical examination under the ADA and thus can be used as a pre-offer selection procedure to determine the qualifications of the applicants for the job opening.

We base this view on the fact that validated employment tests (including personality tests) are designed to be job-related and predictive of job performance. They constitute an effective and efficient way to conduct a pre-employment inquiry about an individual's job-related knowledge, skill, or ability. This position is also consistent with the case law that has been associated with the 1973 Rehabilitation Act (Arnold & Thiemann, 1992). In contrast, medical examinations have a completely different purpose than employment tests. They are designed to be diagnostic of the existence, nature, or severity of a physical or medical condition, and by definition, are impermissible pre-employment inquiries under the ADA. To illustrate, employment tests are intended to measure worker requirements such as "conscientiousness," whereas a diagnostic examination would be intended to develop a diagnosis such as "obsessive compulsive." Employment tests are designed to develop correct inferences regarding the suitability of the individual for a particular job. In contrast, a diagnostic examination is usually the basis of a treatment plan. We hope that the EEOC and the courts will interpret the application of the Act in this manner.

Despite the logic involved, we do take this position somewhat cautiously. This is because psychological tests, especially personality measures, have long been used in the detection and determination of disabilities, as in Social Security disability determinations. Thus, policy makers appear to be concerned with the use of tests of any sort in the screening of applicants with disabilities. In fact, at the time of this writing, there are indications that the EEOC might interpret the use of a test in personnel selection based on it's origin or derivation. In the opinion of some, the use of clinically derived personality inventories (e.g., MMPI) or projective devices (e.g., Miner Sentence Completion test [Miner, 1985]), because of the potential for diagnostic information, may be regarded as a pre-employment medical inquiry. Such devices would then need to be administered post-offer, if at all.

Organizational Entry

Entry as a Mixed Motive Situation

The overview of personnel selection systems offered at the outset of this chapter might lead to the impression that, in well-designed programs, staffing decisions are made by using standard procedures and are carried out with little difficulty. But this would be misleading. In most instances staffing decisions must be formulated with imperfect information. And in all cases they are carried out with the realization that decisions made will affect the lives and careers of individuals (applicants, human resource professionals, managers). Thus it is not surprising that affect and emotions, needs and wants, ideals and pragmatics are involved. The staffing context is indeed a complex venue for implementing the ADA.

Some writers (Porter, Lawler, & Hackman, 1975) have characterized the staffing process as a mixed motive situation. This can be seen from a discussion of at least two points of view—that of the hiring manager and the applicant. The hiring manager typically desires to fill a position promptly. Being able to recruit and hire someone is quite a luxury, especially in the face of corporate restructuring that is so prevalent today. Openings that are not filled in a timely manner might be in jeopardy. Thus, the hiring manager is usually under some pressure to make a decision.

On the other hand, the hiring manager is also concerned with getting the right individual. Although in recent times there are usually many applicants for a given job opening, only a few will be qualified. And in spite of the decision aids available (e.g., tests), experience has shown that it is difficult to assess an applicant's true capabilities. Yet the work unit depends on having an effective person in the position.

The experienced manager also knows that the very qualified applicants are able to get job offers elsewhere. If she or he does not do a good job of quickly identifying who is to be hired and then start actively recruiting (e.g., selling the applicant on the merits of the company), such individuals will soon no longer be available. Moreover, it is common for the manager to be held accountable for promoting greater diversity in the work force. To lose a qualified minority applicant or member of a targeted group to a competing organization would be particularly disconcerting.

Thus the hiring manager feels a cross-current of forces—some inducing care and diligence, others promoting speed. Some motivate directness and candor, others seem to call for putting the "best face forward" when it comes to the benefits of the company and the job.

Theory and research also suggest that the applicant feels a mixture of motives as well. These stem from the competitive nature of organizational entry. This has several implications. Most fundamentally, individuals in a job search seek to present themselves in the best possible light. In the abstract, there are tremendous pressures to do what it takes to preserve a favorable self-image and to seek validation for one's capabilities (Arkin & Sheppard, 1989; Wanous, 1980). This is particularly true in tough economic times where being turned down (rejected) is common. On a strictly practical level, job search is time-consuming, even costly. And after all, the applicant does need a job, the sooner the better. So getting a job becomes a consuming goal. All this ensures that the typical applicant in the selection/screening process is likely to emphasize his/her accomplishments and positive attributes. Any weaknesses are played down or are ignored whenever possible. Clearly disqualifying information is left up to the hiring manager to uncover.

Yet most applicants with any work experience also understand that it is important to get a job that "fits." That is, they want one where their particular set of knowledge, skills, abilities, and interests are relevant. Most individuals do not want the anguish and frustration of failure once on the job. Certainly no one wants the stigma of being fired because they will not or cannot do the work.

For the applicant then, strategic self-presentation must be balanced with candid disclosure. Seeking critical information about the job and its demands may take a back seat to selling oneself. Issues of how open one can be are colored by the fear of being turned down. The job search process is truly a conflictual one.

The Bases for Collaboration

Notice that while both parties characterized above share similar pressures, it is also the case that, in the best of all worlds, both have the same goal. That is to say, ideally, after the hiring decision is made by a manager and the applicant has accepted an offer, they both want to feel good about it. They wish to anticipate a good fit between the demands of the job (worker requirements) and the capabilities and needs of the applicant.

Herein lies a possible common ground. And perhaps this implies a strategy for collaboration. While both parties cannot ignore the competitive nature of most hiring contexts, they need to see that if they can accept the "frame" of the other, they might find ways to work together to ensure that a good fit does occur. The case to be developed in the next section illustrates how this might be done.

When it comes to individuals with disabilities, there is no reason to believe that many of the generalized observations about applicants will also not apply. However, by virtue of their life experiences, there are several other considerations that probably are salient. A recent survey of individuals with disabilities confirms this.

A survey of a sample of readers of the magazine *Careers and the DisAbled* (*Careers*, 1992) revealed that when it comes to gaining organizational entry, they expect employers to have "patience, understanding, and empathy, and not patronize, parent, or pity" (p. 54). For example, one respondent wrote "Never assume that a person with a disability needs help. Instead, just ask what kind of adaptation is necessary...." (p. 54). Another said: "Keep an open mind. Be creative about necessary accommodations.... Treat us as individuals. I only ask for a fair chance to prove that I am able" (pp. 54-55). "Ask about abilities first. Then ask what accommodation would help achieve my maximum potential" (p. 55). And another writes: "Our needs are usually less than what you perceive them to be" (p. 55).

The results of the survey (35.6% response rate) are instructive for other reasons. Survey respondents included college students and professionals from corporations and government agencies. Fifty-nine percent of the sample are mobility impaired. The remainder consists of individuals who are hearing impaired (13.8%); are visually impaired (12.6%); have hidden (e.g., non-visible) disabilities (10.7%) and learning disabilities (3.8%). About 30% of the respondents said that they are unemployed but employable, while 37.5% were full-time working professionals, 10.8% worked part-time. And 22% were full-time college students.

Finally, the respondents of the survey offer a great deal of advice to their peers who might be seeking employment. They include the following suggestions:

- Research the company that you want to work for.

- You must learn to speak up for yourself. Be confident.

- Be up-front with employers about your disability. You need to educate the interviewer to your individual accommodations.

- Be persistent.

- Know your rights under the ADA.

- Discuss accommodations when the time is right and explain that others may benefit from these accommodations.

- Do not expect others to accept the burden of your disability. Only ask for assistance in carrying it yourself.

- You are employed in a job because of your expertise in that area, not for who or what you are. If you are the best, then that cannot be taken away from you. People will see beyond any disabilities or limitations (p. 57).

The results of this survey have been reviewed in some detail in order to amplify on the theme of this section. Our belief is that, while organizational entry is indeed a competitive process, one that produces a variety of cross-currents and mixed motives, with proper framing, applicants with disabilities and employers have ample grounds to work together. More specifically, if the sample of respondents is at all typical of applicants with disabilities, in order to bring about a mutually satisfying placement what will be needed is good will, mutual respect and empathy, appropriate and timely information, a problem solving orientation, and adequate preparation by all of the parties (applicant, staffing specialist, hiring manager) involved. These themes will be developed below.

Accommodation in Action

In our example we will describe an individual with a disability who has applied for a position as a customer service representative in a large financial services company. We will use it to illustrate the application of the ADA to the hiring process from two points of view: the applicant with the disability and the employer. For purposes of this example, we will assume that the applicant has a "hidden" disability. We will also assume that our applicant is "otherwise qualified" (as described in an earlier section of this chapter) based on his previous work experience in a customer contact position for a fast food company. We will also assume that the employer utilizes a comprehensive application process including an application form, structured interviews, employment testing, and reference checks.

Throughout our example, we will highlight reasonable accommodation as it might occur at different points in the hiring process. While selection into an organization is indeed competitive, there will be ample ground for the applicant and the employer to work together. Thus, we will present it as an interactive process requiring communication and flexibility by both parties. In order to understand this interactive process, it is helpful to review some of the general principles that surround the ADA reasonable accommodation obligation.

Reasonable Accommodation

The EEOC lists some basic principles to keep in mind when deciding upon a reasonable accommodation (Americans with Disabilities Act, 1992, III-3 to III-5). These include:

- A reasonable accommodation must be an effective accommodation.

- The reasonable accommodation obligation applies only to accommodations that reduce barriers to employment related to a person's disability.

- A reasonable accommodation need not be the best accommodation available, as long as it is effective for the purpose.

- An employer is not required to provide an accommodation that is primarily for the personal use of the applicant (e.g., wheelchair, artificial limb).

- The ADA's requirements for certain types of adjustments and modifications to meet the reasonable accommodation obligation do not prevent an employer from providing accommodations beyond those required by the ADA.

While the EEOC uses the term "effective," it does not provide clear standards to help in determining whether or not an accommodation is "effective." In our opinion, an effective accommodation in the hiring process is one that meets the legitimate needs of both parties the applicant and the employer. That is, it would be effective if it is acceptable to the applicant with a disability and would enable him/her to participate fairly in the hiring process (i.e., by enabling his/her qualifications to be demonstrated or exhibited). But is also must meet the needs of the employer. In most cases, this means that the accommodation should be logistically and technically feasible and should not violate the integrity of a well-developed selection procedure (i.e., raise issues of validity, reliability, and utility presented in an earlier section of this chapter). It is also important that the accommodation be perceived as fair by members of the general applicant pool as they will frequently be aware of accommodation practices. Finally, it should be "fair" in the context of corporate culture.

Reasonable accommodation in the staffing process usually is determined on the particular facts of the individual case because the nature of the disability and the selection procedure (e.g., employment test) will vary. Both the employer and the applicant have responsibilities here. The EEOC's interpretive guidelines (Americans with Disabilities Act, 1992, Appendix, B-43) suggest a four-step process for determining the most appropriate form of reasonable accommodation. The steps are:

1) Analyze the job and determine its purpose and essential functions;

2) Consult with the individual with the disability to determine the precise job-related limitations and how those limitations could be overcome with a reasonable accommodation;

3) In consultation with the individual to be accommodated, identify potential accommodations and assess the effectiveness of each; and

4) Consider the preference of the individual to be accommodated and select and implement the accommodations that are the most appropriate for the applicant and the employer.

In most cases, the applicant will be one of the best sources for suggesting an appropriate accommodation based on his/her "real life" experiences in managing his/her disability.

The employer's obligation to provide a reasonable accommodation applies only to known physical or mental limitations. Where accommodation is asked for but the basis is not obvious, the employer may want to ask for information to assist in determining whether or not a request is appropriate. The ADA specifically states that an employer may request this documentation. More will be said about this in a case example.

Undue Hardships

An employer may not be required to provide a reasonable accommodation if doing so would impose an undue hardship on the operation of its business. The concept of undue hardship (Americans with Disabilities Act, 1992, III-12) includes any action that is unduly costly, extensive, substantial, disruptive, or that would fundamentally alter the nature of operation of the business.

Whether a particular accommodation will impose an undue hardship will be determined on a case-by-case basis. In general, a larger employer would be expected to make accommodations that require more effort or expense than a smaller employer. If a particular accommodation would impose an undue hardship, an employer should consider whether there are alternative accommodations that would not impose such a hardship; whether there is funding available from another source, such as a state vocational rehabilitation agency; or whether the applicant could provide the accommodation.

Documentation

Finally, an employer should document requests for accommodation including all those that were considered or offered, and the applicant's responses to each accommodation discussed, including reasons given for any rejections of the offered accommodations. If a reasonable accommodation is offered and refused and the applicant is unable to participate in the hiring process, the individual with a disability may be considered not qualified for the job opening. On the other hand, the organization will also find it valuable to have collected this information so that, over time, its staff can learn about the nature of requests and how they have been handled in the past. This will enable it to develop or revise the procedures for handling future requests to ensure fair and consistent treatment of all applicants. More about this "organizational learning" will be mentioned later.

Some employers have found it useful to consider accommodations based on the potential administrative, logistical, and/or technical impact of the accommodation. Thus, they might classify the requests as a Level 1, Level 2, Level 3, etc. accommodation. Figure 4.3 (page 66) illustrates one effort to classify possible requests for testing accommodations based on estimates of impacts on the psychometric properties of a test. This concept was presented as "robustness" in an earlier section of this chapter. The employer can then use this type of classification system for determining what type of accommodation is needed, such as the location, equipment, and/or expertise of the individual required to provide the accommodation, etc. This type of classification system can also assist an employer (such as in our example) in ensuring consistent treatment of individuals with disabilities who apply for openings at different locations.

This is an area of both concern and challenges for selection specialists, as they will need to determine and develop the variety of forms or modalities that will allow for accommodation while still retaining the test's ability to produce correct inferences about what is being measured as well as how accurately it is being measured. According to Tenopyr, et al. (1993, p. 9) "not only could the meaning of test scores be changed, but also the sheer ability to make predictions of future behavior or job performance might be altered."

The Case Example

Our applicant has applied for a position as a customer service representative. Our employer has conducted a job analysis of this position to determine the essential functions of the job as well as the knowledge, skills, abilities, and other characteristics required to do this job (as in Figure 4.2).

While conducting the job analysis, the employer followed the EEOC's recommended approach (Americans with Disabilities Act, 1992, II-19 to II-20) by focusing on the purpose of the job as well as the importance of the various job functions in achieving this purpose. The employer examined the importance of a job function by collecting data about the time spent performing the function, the frequency with which the function is performed, and the consequences of the function not being performed. In addition, the employer was careful not to rely solely on the way each function is currently performed as results or outcomes can be achieved in a variety of ways.

The employer used the job analysis results to develop a job description, a structured interview, and an employment test for cognitive abilities. The job description was then used to develop a job advertisement.

Our applicant saw the job advertisement in the local newspaper. Based on how this advertisement was written as well as his previous experience in a customer contact job, the applicant believed that he was qualified for the job. The applicant was also pleased to see the employer's nondiscrimination statement on the basis of disability in the newspaper ad.

The applicant took his resume to the company's local employment office and asked to apply for the advertised position. The company's employment representative reviewed his resume, determined that he was "otherwise qualified" based on his previous work experience, and asked him to complete an application form that had been reviewed (as described in the previous section) to avoid asking questions about a disability or about the nature or severity of a disability. The company's representative described the company's application process, gave the applicant a brochure describing the company's testing process, and made an appointment for a testing session in two days. The representative was careful to state that the applicant was encouraged to request an accommodation at any point in the application process if he would need some adjustment or change because of a limitation caused by a disability.

Back at his home, our applicant read the testing brochure which described each test in the test battery, gave multiple practice items for each test, and overviewed the testing process. The applicant immediately became concerned with the tests' time limits due to his "hidden" disability (i.e., dyslexia) as he had problems taking timed tests in high school. Because he did not have to take an employment test to get his previous job, he was not sure whether or not the difficulties he had taking timed tests in high school would occur again. Thus while he was concerned about revealing his disability which might work to his disadvantage in the application process, he was also concerned that, without accommodation, he would not be able to perform up to his potential.

The applicant remembered the company representative's statement about requesting an accommodation and noticed the company's statement about requesting accommodations prior to the testing session in the brochure. Because he had been given extra time taking tests in high school due to his disability, he decided that he should call and request this type of accommodation.

The next day, the applicant called the company's representative and told her that he would have trouble taking the company's test battery due to a disability. In the conversation, the company's representative avoided asking about the disability and asked instead what type of accommodation was being requested. The applicant reported that he had difficulty taking a timed test and requested that the time limit be extended.

Because of the type of accommodation requested, the company's representative called the company's testing coordinator to report the request. The testing coordinator asked for basic demographic information (e.g., name, address, phone number, etc.) and arranged a time to call the applicant that afternoon.

The testing coordinator conducted a structured interview by telephone that afternoon and recorded the applicant's responses to specific questions. When asked what about the testing program would cause the applicant difficulty due to a physical or mental impairment, the applicant responded that he had difficulty taking timed tests and that he would need a time extension.

This would fall into Level 2 or Level 3 of the company's classification system (see Figure 4.3). The testing coordinator determined that the company would need documentation from a licensed health care provider. The testing coordinator asked if the applicant had any such existing documentation that could be used. When the applicant replied "no", the testing coordinator arranged to send the company's Testing Accommodation Request Form (Figure 4.4) to be completed by a licensed health care provider. The testing coordinator included a copy of the testing brochure so that the licensed professional would have the necessary information to make an informed judg-

Level 1 Accommodation—no appreciable psychometric impact

- providing individual (rather than group) test administration to allow for one or more of the following:
- extra instruction and practice, a rest break after each test
- assistance in holding and steadying the test booklet and/or turning pages
- recording test answers
- using manually scored vs. scannable tests for greater ink/paper contrast
- providing oversize pencil/writing tool, clip board, magnifier, etc.
- adapting the physical environment (e.g., table height, lighting, etc.)
- moving the testing session to a more accessible (e.g., wheelchair) or distraction-free location
- substituting written-testing session instructions for oral instructions
- enlarging the test print
- providing an interpreter to sign the testing instructions
- extending the time limit for power tests

Level 2 Accommodation—possible psychometric impact

- simplifying test language
- extending the time limit for speeded tests
- administering the test in Braille by a reader or on a computer
- substituting a written test for an oral test or the reverse

Level 3 Accommodation - significant psychometric impact

- waiving one or more tests in a test battery
- evaluating the applicant's ability to perform the essential functions of the job through alternative methods such as:
- structured interviews, previous work experience, education, licenses or certification, job demonstration, consultation with the licensed health care provider.

Figure 4.3 Policy-guided accommodation plan: Classification system for test accommodations.

ment and to provide useful information. The testing coordinator encouraged the applicant to do this as soon as possible since the hiring decision would be made shortly. Recognizing that this sense of urgency might occur for other jobs he would be applying for, the applicant made a mental note to talk to his health care provider in order to have such documentation readily available in the future.

When the Employment Testing Accommodation Request Form (Figure 4.4) was completed and returned, the testing coordinator saw that an accommodation of extended time would be needed on only one of the tests (e.g., computation) in the company's test battery. The licensed health care provider had stated that the applicant could transpose numbers due to the nature of his disability and needed extra time to process the numeric information accurately.

The company testing coordinator called the applicant and offered the accommodation of extending the time limit on the computation test by 50% (i.e., from 5 minutes to 7-1/2 minutes). He was also told that the accommodation would be provided in an individual testing session rather than a group testing session. The company had earlier decided to handle all requests for time extension in this manner based on data from the original validation study used to establish the 5-minute limit, research findings from large test publishers, and conversations with representatives from other large companies with testing programs. The company was also collecting data on its testing accommodations to be used to adjust the 50% time extension in the future if needed.

The applicant agreed to this accommodation as it appeared similar to what had been done in testing sessions in high school and it seemed a reasonable accommodation. He also liked the fact that this would be handled in an individual testing session rather than a large group session so he would not be uncomfortable in front of his peers for being "treated differently." The testing coordinator recorded his agreement and explained that this type of accommodation would need to be provided by one of the company's specially trained ADA test administrators rather than by the local employment representative. The applicant was informed that he would be contacted within 2 days.

The applicant was in fact contacted by the company's ADA test administrator the next day and completed the testing process at one of the company's regional offices the same day. The ADA administrator scored his test and conveyed the results to both the company's testing coordinator (who documented the test administration and the test results) and the local employment representative.

In this example, we do not wish to appear to gloss over the fact that the scores from the applicant were obtained from a test administered in a nontraditional manner (i.e., extra time was given). As we discuss later, applicant scores on tests administered in a nontraditional way still need to be interpreted, especially when there is competition for hiring. In an ideal world, there would be empirical evidence that scores under different forms of administration are, in fact, comparable with regard to valid inferences. This is analogous to having "parallel forms" of a test, where a given score (or percentile score) from either measure can be taken at face value.

However, absent any company-specific data on this matter, a few caveats are in order. At a minimum, the human resource professional should contact the test publisher(s) for guidance on the interpretation or conversion to alternative modalities of the test, based on their research. It still might be wise to ensure that the results of such administrations are interpreted only by a consultant trained in psychometrics or a psychologist.

To continue our example, the local employment representative then called the applicant to inform him that he had met the qualifications on the test and scheduled an interview with the hiring manager. The interview went well. The applicant's responses to the structured interview were informative and persuasive. As is typically the case in staffing for this position, the hiring manager then contacted the previous employer for a reference check. During this call any questions that were asked focused on the applicant's previous responsibilities (also a customer service job) and on job performance. He was careful not to ask anything about a disability. Based on all of the information collected during the staffing process—application material, testing results, interview, and reference checks—he was pleased to offer our applicant the position.

As is the case of all job offers made by this financial services institution, this one was contingent upon passing a drug test designed to uncover evidence of illegal substance use. Our applicant was referred to a clinic for this purpose. As with the other worker requirements, this did not present any problems.

From the applicant's point of view, the experience at organizational entry was a satisfying one. Not only was he thrilled with the offer but was impressed with all the contacts he had with individuals from this company. While he was conscious of his disability, he did not feel "different." This appeared to be a company where he would enjoy working and he looked forward to starting work. All in all, it appeared to be a "good fit."

Notice that the issues of accommodation of the applicant-in-training or in the design of the job itself (areas also covered by the ADA), have not been treated in our case example. This is because the focus of this chapter is on the hiring process. Should our case continue, these issues would have to be discussed at the appropriate time with the successful applicant.

While we have presented an example that resulted in our applicant receiving a job offer, we realize that this may not always be the case. For example, our applicant may not have met the qualifications on the employment tests for the position that he was applying for even with the accommodation of extended time. It is important that an organization think through and prepare for as many outcomes as possible. For instance, many organizations have a retesting policy of 3 or 6 months where applicants who do not meet the qualifications on the employment tests may retest after a 3 or 6 month period. Applicants who do not qualify are informed of this retest interval and are invited to reapply at the end of the required

EMPLOYMENT TESTING ACCOMMODATION REQUEST FORM

Please review the company's testing brochure before completing this form. Please note this form does not request that you identify your disability but rather that you identify the limitations caused by a physical or mental disability and any possible accommodations that you are requesting to complete the employment testing process.

The information requested below will be held strictly confidential and will not be shared with any outside source without your written permission.

_____   _____
Applicant Name (Please Print)   *Social Security Number*

Request for an Accommodation (To be completed by applicant)

After reviewing the company's testing brochure, I have determined that due to a sensory (includes the abilities to hear, to see, and to process information), speaking, or manual skills impairment caused by a physical or mental condition, I cannot perform the following test behaviors.[1] List all test behaviors which you cannot perform. For example, "cannot read standard size print." Please be as specific as possible.

_____

_____

The following accommodation is requested to complete the company's employment tests. Identify any accommodation necessary. For example, "provide tests in larger print." Please be as specific as possible.

_____

_____

_____   _____
Applicant signature   *Date*

Your above request for accommodation in the employment testing process must be certified below by a licensed health care provider.

Certification of Need for Accommodation
(To be completed by a licensed health care provider)

I have reviewed the company's testing brochure and it is my professional opinion that due to the applicant's sensory, speaking, or manual skills impairment caused by a physical or mental condition, he/she should be accommodated in the manner described above.[2]

_____   _____
Licensed Health Care Provider Name (Please Print)   *Professional Title*

_____   _____
Licensed Health Care Provider Signature   *Date Form Completed*

_____   _____
Phone Number   *Date Applicant Last Examined*

Figure 4.4 Documenting requests for accommodation:
Employment Testing Request Form.

waiting period. This type of retesting policy could apply to all testing situations, including those where accommodations have been provided. Incidentally, this "reconsideration opportunity" has been found to be an important feature of selection systems that promote the feeling of fairness or procedure justice (Gilliland, in press).

Similarly, our applicant may not have met the qualifications for the position that he was applying for but may have met the qualifications for another open position in the company. In this case, the organization may have developed procedures to forwarding and tracking his application for this open position for ensure that our applicant has access to equal employment opportunities based on merit. Whatever the situation, it is important that the organization be as prepared as possible to handle it. The prudent consultant or human resource professional is the one who will help the organization be prepared for a variety of outcomes.

While this is a contrived example, it is offered as a means of presenting the interactive process requiring communication and flexibility by both parties. We purposely chose a "hidden" disability in order to demonstrate that it is not unreasonable for an employer to request documentation when it is difficult to determine when an accommodation is needed and what is an appropriate accommodation to offer. While most employers are eager "to do the right thing" when dealing with individuals with disabilities in competitive employment situations, they have also learned (often painfully) that there are those who will seek to improve their chances of success, regardless of the means. The challenge is to distinguish between the applicant who truly needs an accommodation in order to compete fairly for a position and the applicant who does not.

We also illustrated the way that an important part of the assessment process, a test battery, was modified in light of a request for accommodation. Note that the test in the battery that was felt to be a problem was not dropped. Instead, its time limits were adjusted in a way that (in this case) still preserved the validity of the measure for people with this disability.

On the other side of the coin, we have the applicant who truly wants to be productive in a meaningful job. Yet, he may need assistance in helping to display his capacities in a competitive situation. He may also bring "baggage" from previous experiences, particularly where he may have failed or lost out due to stereotypes regarding his disability. Thus he needs to be willing to take a risk by self-identifying so that the necessary modifications or changes in the application process can be identified and provided. This is only likely in a comfortable environment. His decision proved to be a good one. Not only was his request honored, he ultimately was offered and accepted the job.

Recap

Throughout this case example, we attempted to illustrate several themes that we feel are important to the successful implementation of the ADA in the staffing process. The first is good will. Organizations must be committed to the spirit of the ADA to make it work well. This must involve all levels of management and be reflected in staffing policies and practices that project support for applicants with disabilities. By initiating the good-will effort with the candidate through sensitivity to his needs and respect for the ADA, we expect that the candidate would be more likely to respond in kind. The fact that the employer is proactive with the good-will effort would help produce a nondefensive response.

A related theme is mutual respect. Representatives of an organization must treat applicants with disabilities as individuals, not members of a class. There is no room for stereotyped thinking. There is a lot of room for listening to the particular needs for accommodation expressed. In turn, applicants with disabilities need to be educated to the legitimate needs and goals of the organization. Applicants of all types must understand that personnel selection is an important activity for most companies, the results of which will affect its future competitiveness. Organizational communications to the public in the context of recruiting can be clear on the importance of the selection process to the organization.

Still another theme is timely information. In our case example, the organization attempted to clearly characterize the nature of the selection/screening process to all applicants early in the relationship. Similarly, the applicant let the organization know of his needs in a timely manner as well. This early exchange of information, when coupled with a problem-solving orientation, produced an effective accommodation. The applicant was explicit with regard to the elements of the staffing process that would create a problem (the timed test). The employer looked for ways that would deal with the problem while still retaining the integrity of the assessment battery.

Finally, both parties need adequate preparation. It is recommended that the employer have clear policies, trained personnel, the private spaces for administration, the empirical evidence of a test's robustness (and/or the range of accommodations/modalities within which it would still be valid), and individuals empowered to make decisions in a timely manner. Similarly, the applicant with a disability must have a realistic self-assessment of his/her job relevant capabilities, understand where and when accommodation might be appropriate in the staffing process, and know just what kind of accommodation is required to exhibit his/her potential. As we illustrated in our case, it is also a good idea for the applicant to have appropriate documentation that might support a request for accommodation available at the outset of the job search process.

Applicant preparation notwithstanding, we do recognize that some applicants with disabilities may still be reluctant to discuss their needs for accommodation because of past discrimination or a fear of being stigmatized. For example, when a person has a mental illness well-controlled by medication. Such individuals should be reassured by the organization that they are not at risk by requesting accommodation. This can be done by having materials clearly stating the company's commitment to their fair treatment, by following good professional practices (as outlined here), and ideally, by being able to point to success stories of qualified individuals with disabilities who have been hired by the company in the past.

In summary, these themes are likely to produce experiences where both the applicant and the employer feel that they can succeed in producing a mutually satisfying job placement.

Problematic Issues

This chapter has been written in an attempt to capture the nature of the likely impact of the ADA on the hiring process. While we have made use of the technical and practitioner literature whenever possible, the fact is, only with time will we be able to determine the law's actual impact. Indeed, some would argue that the ADA raises more issues than it resolves. It will take some years of experience with the law to fully understand its impact. There is some merit in this view. In its goal to ensure access to employment opportunities to individuals with disabilities, the Act often leaves open the question of how best to do this. After thinking about issues of implementation, we have identified the following as particularly problematic:

Employer-Related Issues

a) How many people will seek accommodation under the Act? Estimates of the number of people with disabilities vary greatly, from 15 to 43 million (Blanck, 1992). How many will seek accommodation under the Act? What is the nature of the requests that will be made? What level of successful placement of qualified individuals with disabilities should we expect if all parties are working toward this goal? The answer to these questions will derive in part from how one defines "disability" and what constitutes a "qualified person." Employers have been concerned that they will be overwhelmed with requests for accommodation. Experience to date would seem otherwise. For example, the Ohio Board of Bar Examiners received 24 requests for accommodation in the taking of the 1992 Ohio Bar exam (out of over 5200 applicants). Twelve cases involved vision impairments, six were based on limited use of the hands, one had a back injury. Two candidates reported learning disabilities. Interestingly, two applicants who were pregnant at the time (a condition not covered by the ADA), at their request, were allowed to sit at the back of the hall, a location close to the rest rooms. The accommodations agreed to for the other applicants were equally straightforward (Somerson, 1993).

b) How does an organization create a climate of trust in a nominally competitive context? Individuals with disabilities can report many instances of discrimination in employment contexts. It is understandable that they may approach the staffing process warily and with distrust. On the other hand, staffing specialists can readily document instances where applicants will attempt to misrepresent their qualifications. When trying to build mutual respect and a problem-solving atmosphere, something really needed under the ADA, such cynicism by both parties will continue to be a barrier.

c) What kind of documentation/evidence will be required to demonstrate that an organization is in compliance with the ADA? Most writers on the topic (e.g., Potter & Reesman; 1990) seem to feel that traditional statistical evidence used in Civil Rights cases (e.g., pass rates of protected subgroups) is not appropriate. This view is based on both the language and intent of the Act. Individuals with disabilities are to be treated as unique cases. They are not to be sorted into categories (e.g., sensory impaired, mobility impaired, manually impaired). Thus, group-level statistics, needed for statistical analysis, will not be available. On the other hand, it's not clear just what evidence would be compelling enough to make or refute a charge of unfair discrimination against an individual with a disability.

d) What is the role for personality and trait assessments in the hiring process under the ADA? As pointed out in an earlier section, at this time it is not clear how the EEOC will interpret such tests and procedures designed to measure personal traits or attributes in light of the ADA prohibition on pre-offer medical inquiries. Our position is that the use of valid psychological assessment procedures designed to measure the personal qualities—including personality or emotional characteristics—necessary for job performance, when they are bonafide occupational requirements, is consistent with the intent of the ADA. It also appears to be supported by case law (Arnold & Thiemann, 1992). Moreover, while the evidence for the utility of any selection device must guide any decision regarding its appropriateness in a particular context, we would not like to see whole classes of potentially useful decision aids (e.g., personality measures) be ruled out unilaterally. It is unfortunate that this controversy comes at a time when staffing specialists are becoming more impressed with personality measures as they have been able to contribute to the prediction of job success in several settings (Barrick & Mount, 1991).

To have job-relevant personality assessments available before making an offer, is not only logical but may be cost-effective. The employer is then able to use valuable data where it is needed to make selection decisions.

e) What is the obligation of the organization to contribute to the vocational rehabilitation and gainful employment of individuals with disabilities? Various interpretations of the Act (e.g., Blanck, 1992) place more or less of a burden on private companies in this regard. On the face of it, the Act does not require a company to hire a person with a disability who is not qualified. On the other hand, it also appears that in some cases, what is meant by an "essential function" of a job is left ambiguous. This shows up in how the ADA defines what does or does not constitute "undue hardship." To the point, in addition to cost, "undue hardship" is related to the capacity of the hiring organization to redefine the essential duties of a job. For example, in the instance of hiring employees to perform a given job in a company, it is presumed to be less of a burden (e.g., makes accommodation more feasible) if some duties that would normally have to be carried out by an applicant with a disability are instead assigned to others.

Given modern technology (e.g., computers as interfaces) and appropriate financing, it is possible to redesign any job to the level of the capacities of almost any applicant. That is to say, through some combination of accommodation/job redesign, a viable employment situation for any individual with a disability can be created (see Blanck's [1992] analysis regarding how this might work in the case of an individual with severe mental retardation). To put it another way, does the Act promote a placement (rather than a selection) model of staffing? In some respects, it can be interpreted this way, whereby an organization is expected to match up a motivated individual with a disability to any number of job openings that vary in their essential functions (and hence, worker requirements) until a suitable match can be found. If this position were to be adopted, it might imply that staffing specialists in the future would be wise to make use of assessment methods and technology designed for effective and efficient placement, as developed by researchers and practitioners in the military (e.g., Wiskoff & Rampton, 1989).

f) To what extent must the attitudes of managers and staffing specialists be changed in order to successfully implement the Act? From a logistical standpoint, managers and staffing specialists will need to have patience with the new process, because to do it correctly will necessarily take slightly longer to hire someone (in many cases). Managers and staffing specialists will need to refrain from cutting corners to fill slots quickly. Organizations will need to be sensitive to any pressure being put on these people to give quicker results. Not conducting the process correctly and succumbing to pressure only defeats the purpose of ADA.

On a more technical level, the need for attitude shifts relate to the widespread norm (some skeptics might say "myth") of selection by merit in American society. For the most part, many individuals think in terms of getting the very best person for the job out of a pool of qualified individuals. Their selection models are thus of the "top down" variety. That is to say, after rank ordering the applicants in terms of qualifications, job offers are first made to those at the top of the list. This strategy is followed in the belief that there are demonstrable benefits to both the individual and the organization to hire the most qualified person (see labor economists' reference to "human capital," Becker, 1974). On the other hand, the ADA regularly makes reference to the "qualified applicant with a disability." Some have interpreted this to mean that the framers of the Act were thinking of only two classes of people—those who are and are not (at least minimally) qualified for a job. Thus, as long as the applicant meets certain minimal (but acceptable) criteria he or she is protected under the Act. If this is indeed the case, the act and prevailing practices are at odds with one another. This may only be clarified through litigation. But there should be better ways to resolve the issue.

Applicant-Related Issues

g) How to ensure realistic self-knowledge on the part of applicants with a disability? This is not an issue just for individuals with disabilities. In fact, many job candidates appear to have an enhanced (and often unrealistic) image of their capabilities and potential (Wanous, 1980). However, for individuals with disabilities, it would seem to be especially important to have a clear understanding of the types of accommodations needed. This will help to ensure that an accommodation is requested only when it is needed and that the accommodation provided will be appropriate. Going through a staffing process without requesting accommodation when it is truly needed, helps no one. The applicant may fail to perform up to his/her true capabilities.

The issue of self-assessment might be especially complex for cases where an individual is newly disabled and seeks to come back to work. Knowledge of the capacity to perform, with or without accommodation, may be uncertain. Any accommodation requests may, in fact, be based on little more than intuition.

How might realistic self-knowledge be enhanced? Clearly, the individual has some obligation in this regard. Seeking out valid feedback and counsel from friends and rehabilitation specialists would help. Making use of professional and specialist networks would also seem appropriate (e.g., Job Accommodation Network). However, there is no substitute for diligence and homework. When it comes to applying for particular jobs and/or for preparing for the selection process itself, it will be very helpful to really understand the physical, mental and emotional demands of both. Deep knowledge of the selection process in particular, can allow for critical self-assessment and for the mental, logistical, and even physical preparation needed to do well. Such homework can involve contacting current employees, search firms and human resource specialists used by the company.

We have already alluded to the role that the company itself may play in encouraging a good match between the applicant with a disability and the organization. However, it is worth repeating that a careful job analysis and an accurate public portrayal of both the position in question and the hiring process in particular will go a long way to assist the applicant in a self-assessment. It would also be useful to have a company ADA coordinator available and ready to discuss applicant questions. On a more progressive level, organizations might offer orientation sessions to prospective applicants with disabilities. With no commitment implied for any party, such individuals would then experience (and thus more validly choose and prepare for) the process of going through the organization's selection system. This more progressive approach has been used successfully to encourage underrepresented groups (e.g., women) to apply for and succeed in achieving job placements in traditionally ignored career areas (e.g., skilled trades, police, and safety work). It might work well here as well.

h) What is the role of "third parties" in assisting the applicant in the selection process? Under what conditions should a friend, personal reader, or job coach be asked to assist in the assessment process? Who is the best party to turn to in order to obtain the requested documentation? Whose advice should be sought to choose the type of accommodation that is required? How can the role of third parties (ombudsman, mediator) be legitimized so as to reduce or minimize disputes, disputes that might otherwise lead to litigation?.

Technical/Psychometric Issues

i) How do various requests for accommodation in test format or modality affect key properties of the selection systems, notably validity and utility? While one would normally think that this is an empirical question, there are several factors contributing to making simple empirical solutions problematic. One is the likelihood of highly individualized accommodation requests. This implies a large number of potentially different forms of administration and hence small samples in any one form to work with. Another is that established procedures for equating tests are difficult to apply in the case of individuals with disabilities.

Under normal circumstances, equating two forms of a test involves using two groups of individuals selected and assigned at random to take each version. Performance levels and other psychometric indices (e.g., equal standard deviations, distributions) are then reviewed for comparability. Even if they are not, the procedure allows for the calibration/transformation of scores. However, in the case of disabled individuals, where the groups are pre-chosen, the controls implied by random assignment are missing. An alternative approach, one that relies on the performance or matching on anchor tests may offer some possibilities. But here also it would be necessary to assume that performance on the anchor is itself not influenced by the nature of the impairment (Tenopyr et al., 1993).

However an alternative form of a test or selection device is created, it will be important to assess its operating characteristics relative to the standards outlined earlier. To the extent that this is established, we could say that the assessment tool in its new modality or format is defensible from a professional point of view.

j) Related to the point just made, how should one interpret scores derived from the nonstandard administration of selection devices? How meaningful are such scores for making appropriate inferences? Are adjusted scores actually worse than the alternative of dropping the challenged element of a selection battery from the information that would be available from a candidate? Do modifications in administration unfairly advantage certain applicants?

Professional standards (e.g., those of APA or the Society for Industrial/Organizational Psychology) typically call for investigation of the meaning of scores derived from tests when administration conditions differ. This refers to its construct validity (Messick, 1989). There are ample logical grounds to argue that changing the modality of administration or the timing of the test will greatly alter the construct being assessed. The meaning of scores can be assessed in light of its predictive validity. But here again, the key assumptions must be made that performance on a criterion measure (e.g., job performance), is itself unaffected by a disability. Work done on the Scholastic Aptitude Test and the Graduate Record Exam (e.g., Willingham, 1988, as cited in Tenopyr et al., 1993) is encouraging, however. Comparable reliability and item difficulties have been reported for groups of individuals with different types of disabilities. But the predictive validity evidence obtained in an academic context does show that modified tests can lead to both under- and over-prediction, depending on the type of disability involved and the kind of accommodation used (see also Nester, in press). Once again, a major factor hampering research is the relatively small number of cases available to study. Some of the samples were as small as 35 for modified tests administered to those with visual impairments (Tenopyr et al., 1993).

This concern for the meaning of tests administered in non standard ways extends to how and under what conditions scores should be "flagged." The flagging or tagging of scores is a common practice used to inform the reader that they should not be taken at face value. But the flagging of scores in the context of the ADA raises legal, ethical, and practical issues as well (Tenopyr et al., 1993). Certainly those doing research with test scores would need a record of which ones are associated with modified tests and procedures. Similarly, we also feel that organizations will need such information in order to learn from their experiences with accommodation as to what works to meet the needs of applicants with disabilities. On the other hand, there are legal questions as to how much information about nonstandard administration should be made available to managers, even when well motivated, since a flagged score would reveal that an applicant or a new employee has a disability, where this might not be otherwise obvious (e.g., a hidden disability). To some this might violate the letter of the ADA. Knowledge that the practice of flagging of scores exists also might serve to dissuade some individuals with disabilities from asking for accommodations. This would certainly violate the spirit of the ADA.

Each of these areas represent challenges to the successful implementation of the ADA in the context of staffing organizations. On the other hand, each also can be viewed as a venue for research and development. In varying degrees, the issues raised lend themselves to empirical work. While we do not have the space to outline how this might be done, we hope that the content of this chapter might provide enough guidance to start the efforts in this direction.

A Call For Organizational Learning

The implementation of the ADA may indeed be a challenge for some organizations. In order to best meet this challenge it will be important for managers and staffing specialists in organizations to take every opportunity to learn from their own and other's experiences. In our case example, we stressed the possibility of documenting both the nature of the requests for accommodation and the type of accommodation agreed upon. Such information if summarized carefully, can become the basis for inferring certain patterns and trends. These, in turn, could be used to guide future requests for accommodation. Thus any normative requests for accommodation (those within certain parameters) could be handled routinely. Moreover, if such data were integrated with a candidate's performance on the selection device in question, and, ideally, with levels of performance on the job, much could be learned. Insights regarding the impact (if any) of various accommodations (or classes of accommodation) might be determined.

What we are calling for here is a type of organizational learning. One that is based on the careful recording of cases. It is learning that is built on a number of particular, similar (but never identical) instances. The capacity for such learning requires the design and development of staffing processes or routines, a well-conceived and implemented information system, trained (and motivated) personnel, and the regular use of feedback procedures (Fiol & Lyles, 1985; Walsh & Ungson, 1991). It also helps to have an "internal champion" with the capacity (power/resources) to keep such systems in order and operating as intended.

Organizational learning also implies working with other companies to discover what their experiences have been. While information on applicant flows and on accommodation requests and occurrences could be viewed as proprietary, we feel that it is in the best interests of all parties interested in the implementation of the ADA to work together. Many models for inter-organizational cooperation exist here. Industry trade groups, consortia, professional networks (e.g., Job Accommodation Network), etc., have all been used in the past as vehicles for developing data bases and for the dissemination of information or insights that would benefit a particular industry as a whole. Moreover, in the U.S. today, it is increasingly common for organizations to use the concept of "benchmarking" to isolate world-class standards in a way that might be used to guide policy and practice. Just what benchmarks might be identified to reference exemplary efforts in the context of hiring of qualified individuals with disabilities? In fact, why can't the implementation of the ADA be positioned as part of a TQM effort? Similarly, organizations increasingly rely on research into corporate "best practices" as well. What all these efforts have in common is that they can be used as the basis for additional organizational learning (albeit vicarious). We recommend that research be undertaken to see if some of these can be incorporated into efforts to learn about the best ways to implement the ADA.

Finally, organizational learning implies working with other strategic partners to profit from experience. These include test developers and publishers (e.g., ETS) who are in an excellent position to create the large samples needed for research on the effects that different forms of modification might have on selection devices. And most certainly, alliances must be struck with those public and private agencies that are involved in providing rehabilitation, training, and other services to individuals with disabilities. With the cooperation of these entities, a great deal of insight regarding the best staffing policies and practices under the ADA can be uncovered.

In closing, it must be clear by now that in our judgment, it is not sufficient to have the desire or the will to implement the ADA. Good faith efforts are not enough. The progressive organization must have key processes and systems for learning in place in order to be successful in moving from following the letter of the law to implementing its spirit.

Editors' Notes

[1,2] Although this wording is based on the language in the EEOC regulation, there are differences of opinion regarding its interpretation of the law's intent. The reader is advised to seek legal counsel before adopting any specific phrases for a form of this sort.

References

Americans with Disabilities Act. (1992). *Technical assistance manual on the employment provisions* (Title I). Washington, DC: Equal Employment Opportunity Commission.

Anderson, C. D., Warren, J. L., & Spencer, C. C. (1984). Inflation bias in self-assessment examinations: Implications for valid employee selection. *Journal of Applied Psychology, 69,* 574–580.

Arkin, R. M., & Sheppard, J. A. (1989). Self presentation styles in organizations. In R. Giacabone & P. Rosenfeld (Eds.), *Impression management in the organization.* Hillsdale, NJ: Lawrence Erlbaum.

Arnold, D. W., & Thiemann, A. J. (1992). To test or not to test: The status of psychological testing under the ADA. *Criminal Justice Digest, 11,* 13.

Arvey, R. D., & Faley, R. H. (1981). *Fairness in selecting employees.* (2nd Ed.). Reading, MA: Addison Wesley.

Barrick, M. R., & Mount, M. K. (1991). The big five personality dimensions and job performance: A meta analysis. *Personnel Psychology, 44,* 1–26.

Blanck, P. D. (1992). Empirical study of the employment provisions of the Americans with Disabilities Act: Methods, preliminary findings and implementations. *New Mexico Law Review, 22,* 1, 120–241.

Blumberg, M., & Pringle, C. D. (1982). The missing opportunity in organizational research: Some implications for a theory of work performance. *Academy of Management Review, 7*, 560–569.

Brinberg, D., & McGrath, J. E. (1982). A network of validity concepts within the research process. In D. Brinberg & L. Kidder (Eds.), *New directions for methodology of social and behavioral science: Forms of validity in research* (No. 12). San Francisco: Jossey-Bass.

Campbell, D. T. (1969). Reforms as experiments. *American Psychologist, 24*, 4, 409–429.

Campion, M. A., Pursell, E., & Brown, B. K. (1988). Structured interviewing: Raising the psychometric properties of the employment interview. *Personnel Psychology, 41*, 1, 25–52.

Careers and the DisAbled. (1992). Second annual readers survey. pp. 54–51.

Cascio, W. F. (1992). *Costing human resources: The financial impact of behavior in organizations.* Boston: Kent.

Evans, B. R. (December 1992). Will employees and unions cooperate? *H.R. Magazine,* pp. 59–76.

Feldblum, C. R. (1991). Employment protections. In J. West, (Ed.), *The Americans with Disabilities Act: From policy to practice.* (pp. 81–110). NY: Milbank McCarrol Fund.

Fiol, C. M., & Lyles, M. A. (1985). Organizational learning. *Academy of Management Review, 10*, 4, 803–813.

Fitz-Enz, J. (1984). *How to measure human resources management.* New York: McGraw-Hill.

Fowler, E. M. (1990). Careers: Personnel executives on the rise. *New York Times,* May 9.

Gael, S. (Ed.). (1987). *Job analysis handbook.* New York: Wiley.

Gilliland, S. W. (in press). Perceived fairness of selection systems: An organizational justice perspective. *Academy of Management Review.*

Kane, M.T. (1992). An argument-based approach to validity. *Psychological Bulletin, 112*, 3, 527–535.

Katzell, R., & Austin, J. A. (1992). From then to now: The development of industrial/organizational psychology in the United States. *Journal of Applied Psychology, 77*, 6, 803–835.

Landy, F. J. (1986). Stamp collecting vs. science: Validation as hypothesis testing, *American Psychologist, 41*, 1183–1192.

Levine, E. L. (1983). *Everything that you always wanted to know about job analysis.* Tampa, FL: Mariner Press.

Messick, S. (1989). Validity. In Robert L. Linn (Ed.). *Educational measurement,* (pp. 13–103). Macmillan.

Miner, J. B. (1985). Sentence completion measures in personnel research. The development and validation of the Miner Sentence Completion Scales. In H. J. Bernandin & D. A. Bownas (Eds.), *Personality assessment in organizations.* (pp. 145–176). New York: Praeger.

Munsterberg, H. (1913). *Psychology and industrial efficiency.* Boston: Houghton-Mifflin.

Nester, M. A. (in press). Psychometric testing and reasonable accommodation for persons with disabilities. *Rehabilitation Psychology.*

Potter, E. E., & Reesman, A. E. (1990). *The Americans with Disabilities Act: Testing and other employee selection procedures.* Washington DC: National Foundation for the Study of Employment Policy.

Porter, L. W., Lawler, E. E. III, & Hackman, J. R. (1975). *Behavior in organizations.* NY: McGraw-Hill.

Reilly, R. R., & Chao, G. T. (1982). Validity and fairness of some alternative employee selection procedures. *Personnel Psychology, 35,* 1–62.

Rynes, S. L., & Barber, A. E. (1990). Applicant attraction strategies: An organizational perspective. *Academy of Management Review, 15,* 286–310.

Schmidt, F. L., Hunter, J. E., & Pearlman, K. (1982). Assessing the economic impact of personnel programs on workforce productivity. *Personnel Psychology, 35,* 333–347.

Schmidt, F. L., & Hunter, J. E. (1981). Employment testing: Old theory and new research findings. *American Psychologist, 36,* 1128–1137.

Schmidt, F. L., Hunter, J. E., McKenzie, R. C., & Muldrow, T. N. (1979). Impact of valid selection procedures on workforce productivity. *Journal of Applied Psychology, 64,* 609–626.

Schmitt, N., & Borman, W. C. (1993). *Personnel selection in organizations.* San Francisco: Jossey-Bass.

Schmitt, N., & Landy, F. J. (1992). The concept of validity. In N. Schmitt, & W. Borman, (Eds.), *Personnel selection in organizations,* San Francisco: Jossey-Bass.

Schmitt, N., & Klimoski, R. J. (1991). *Research methods in human resources management.* Cincinnati, OH: South-Western.

Schmitt, N., Gooding, R. Z., Noe, R. A., and Kirsch, M. (1984). Meta-analysis of validity studies published between 1964–1982 and an investigation of study characteristics. *Personnel Psychology. 37*, 407–422.

Scott, W. D. (1911). *Increasing human efficiency in business.* NY: Macmillan.

Segal, J. A. (December 1992). Drugs, alcohol, and the ADA. *HR Magazine,* pp. 73–76.

Spencer, L. M. Jr., (1986). *Calculating human resource cost and benefits: Cutting costs and improving productivity.* New York: Wiley.

Somerson, M. D. (Jan. 8, 1993). Learning disabled can step up to bar. *Columbus (OH) Dispatch.*

Tenopyr, M. L., Angoff, W. H., Butcher, J. N., Geisinger, K. F., & Reilly, R. R. (1993). Psychometric and assessment issues raised by the Americans with Disabilities Act (ADA). *The score, XV, 4,* 1–15.

Walsh, J. P., & Ungson, G. R. (1991). Organizational memory. *Academy of Management* . Review, 16, 1, 57–91.

Wanous, J. P. (1980). *Organizational entry: Recruitment, selection, socialization of newcomers.* Reading, MA: Addison Wesley.

Willingham, W. W. (1988). Testing handicapped people—the validity issue. In H. Wainer & H. Braun (Eds.), *Test validity* (pp. 89–103). Hillsdale, NJ: Lawrence Erlbaum Assoc.

Wiskoff, M. F., & Rampton, G. M. (1989). *Military personnel measurement, testing, assignment, evaluation.* New York: Praeger.

· 5 ·

The Americans with Disabilities Act and Individuals with Neurological Impairments

Paul R. Sachs and Cathy A. Redd

The Americans with Disabilities Act (ADA) protects individuals with physical and mental disabilities in their pursuit of vocational options that are so essential to independent living (Equal Employment Opportunity Commission & Department of Justice, 1991; EEOC, 1992). The ADA also has an affect on the activities of the rehabilitation psychologist who works with such individuals.

The rehabilitation psychologist is in an excellent position to educate and assist employees and employers in developing solutions to problems that may be encountered in employment of individuals with disabilities. The psychologist's expertise in communication, analysis of motivation, negotiation, and conflict resolution is a tremendous asset to the employment process.

This chapter will describe some of the implications of the ADA and the opportunities afforded to the rehabilitation psychologist who works specifically with individuals who have neurological impairments. The emphasis here on individuals with neurological impairments is not gratuitous. These individuals have marked limitations in their ability to re-enter the work force after the onset of their impairment (Cook, 1992; Yeas, 1991). Moreover, they present a combination of physical and cognitive impairments that pose particular difficulties in applying the regulations of the ADA.

It is beyond the scope of this chapter, however, to describe the various difficulties presented by individuals with neurological impairments. Rather, we will discuss general guidelines for vocational rehabilitation work with such individuals in light of the ADA. Our focus is on individuals with those conditions that lead to cognitive impairment. They constitute a diverse group that includes individuals with traumatic brain injury, cerebral infarct, epilepsy, Parkinson's disease, multiple sclerosis, cerebral palsy, and various dementias, among other conditions. Individuals with neurological conditions that do not generally lead to cognitive impairments (e.g., traumatic spinal cord injury or Guillian Barre) will not be a focus of this chapter.

Overview of Neurological Impairments

Although we will not focus on the details of different neurological conditions, several common factors are worthy of consideration in vocational planning and intervention.

Epidemiology

The demographic characteristics of the individuals with neurological impairment must be considered in evaluating the individual's vocational potential. These vary widely. Individuals with congenital or childhood onset neurological conditions such as some cerebral palsy or seizure disorders, must face the limitations imposed by these problems before they enter the workforce. Survivors of traumatic brain injury are largely young adults who are at an early stage in their career development. Multiple sclerosis may affect younger and older adults who are in various stages of their career development. Alzheimer's disease and cerebral infarcts affect an older population, many of whom are retired or are considering retirement.

Cognitive and emotional sequelae

Individuals with neurological impairments present with a combination of cognitive and emotional changes as the result of the neurological condition. Indeed, there is a close interaction between the cognitive and emotional changes as they affect observable behavior. Thus, an individual's difficulties in performing complex job tasks, learning new tasks, and handling the emotional and social demands of work are obstacles to vocational integration.

Moreover, individuals will vary widely in their degree of impairment. Disturbed vocational capacities are easily seen in cases of severe injury or illness. In minor traumatic brain injury (TBI), early stage Alzheimer's disease, or multiple sclerosis, the difficulties are subtle and often difficult to differentiate from the individual's premorbid cognitive and emotional style.

Course of the condition

Neurological conditions may be progressive or static. The complexity of these conditions makes recovery difficult to predict. Thus, the proper timing of vocational intervention for individuals with such conditions is difficult to judge.

The Rehabilitation Psychologist's Role in
the Employment Process

In this section we will address the types of interventions the rehabilitation psychologist provides to persons with neurological impairments and to employers of such individuals in light of the ADA. In addition to describing some general considerations for the psychologist, we will provide detailed case examples that illustrate some difficulties posed in developing interventions for individuals with neurological impairments. These case examples are composites of actual clinical situations. Three general stages of intervention will be discussed: prevocational assessment, vocational placement, and on-the-job interventions.

Prevocational Assessment

Evaluating a person's ability or suitability for a job usually involves an interview and the administration of a battery of vocational interest, aptitude, and cognitive tests. Based on the person's areas of cognitive strength or weakness, and vocational aptitudes and preferences, the psychologist advises the client on vocational options.

In the context of the ADA, the rehabilitation psychologist working with individuals who have neurological impairments must go beyond this traditional approach. The ADA defines disability as the result of a physical or mental impairment. This impairment is separate from the environmental or personality factors that affect the person's functioning. Therefore the psychologist must attempt to document the presence of cognitive and emotional difficulties and differentiate these difficulties from personality or environmental factors as they contribute to the individual's performance on the tests administered. For example, an individual's abrupt, impulsive manner of interacting with others may be the result of a certain pre-existing personality style. It may also, however, be a result of a neurological condition in which cognitive and emotional changes interfere with the individual's ability to monitor verbalizations, or the ability to express smooth motor behavior. These neurologically based changes lead to behavior that gives an observer the impression that the person is abrupt or impulsive.

Many cognitive impairments will not be evident unless elicited by certain environmental conditions. An individual may perform well on a task within the controlled environment of the psychologist's office and yet have difficulty enacting the same behavior within the work environment where there are greatly increased and varied sources of distraction and stimulation. For example, a person may show unimpaired or mildly impaired performance on a memory test during the assessment, but report greatly disrupted memory functioning at home or on the job.

In addition, the psychologist must consider the past history of the individual with premorbid capabilities in an attempt to determine the presence of impairment. For example, poor performance on language tests would be interpreted differently in an individual with a history of low academic performance in language arts and a job that involved nonverbal skills, such as mechanical or construction work, than would the same performance in an individual with a history of strong language skills and work in a similar area, such as teaching or practicing law.

The history of the individual's experiences in social and work situations is also important because the person may be protected under the ADA if he/she has a history of a disability whether or not he/she is currently limited by it. For example, an individual who has been diagnosed with multiple sclerosis and was impaired by the condition in the past, but is not currently substantially limited by the condition, would be protected by the ADA.

Combinations of difficulties may be considered an impairment even though the individual difficulties considered alone do not obstruct the individual in life activities. For example, a client with a mild traumatic brain injury may have relatively minor difficulties with attention, concentration, and memory. Furthermore, the person may be able to perform the isolated aspects of jobs such as answering the phone, participating in a business meeting, and writing out policies and procedures. Jobs, however, are rarely so discretely organized. Most likely, the individual has to shift from one task to another, often performing several different tasks in rapid succession. Taking these tasks and cognitive impairments together, the individual could be considered impaired in the ability to perform the job as a whole.

Assessment must consider the nature and severity of the impairment; only those considered long-term or permanent would require the employer to make accommodations for the individual as put forth in the ADA. Prognosis for some conditions is difficult to judge and improvements may occur over a period of years as the individual adapts to injury and receives rehabilitative care. To enhance the ability to judge the client's prognosis, the rehabilitation psychologist should seek historical information about the client's development and work/school performance, carefully examine the client's actual test performance, and attempt to understand the client's test scores in the context of actual life activities. Sometimes, follow-up testing of the client can determine if there is a trend toward further improvement or deterioration in cognitive functioning that would bear out the question of permanence of impairment.

Case Example

C. L. is a 54-year-old married man who experienced a cerebral infarct while on the job as a pipe fitter for a general contracting firm. He had a one-week stay in a rehabilitation hospital and outpatient treatment. He complained of headaches, difficulties in concentration, and word-finding. His wife reported that he occasionally lost track of what he was doing when he was around the house. She noted that his behavior was inconsistent—on some days very confused and fatigued, and on others quite alert and active. Psychological testing performed at the conclusion of his outpatient treatment showed generally unimpaired performance with the exception of slowed motor speed, reduced speech intelligibility, and some word-finding difficulties.

C. L. was intensely motivated to return to work. He felt that he would continue to improve, and eventually be able to return to full work capacity. The psychologist, however, questioned C.L.'s endurance and ability to perform his previous work duties. It was felt that he would not be able to manage some of the planning and decision-making aspects of his job.

To further assess his suitability to return to work, the psychologist and an occupational therapist visited a construction site in order to observe the types of work C. L. would need to perform. Work activities were simulated in the outpatient setting. C. L. performed some of the skills, but also showed more speed and reasoning problems than were evident on formal psychological testing. The simulated activities were performed over a period of days enabling the psychologist to observe C. L.'s inconsistency in performance. Portions of the simulation were videotaped for use within the outpatient setting but not released to C. L.'s employer. The psychologist and C. L. reviewed the videotape and discussed the difficulties that C. L. would face in returning to his previous position. They also discussed some ways in which C. L. could perform some work activities that were within his capabilities, and how these might be modified to accommodate his disabilities.

This example illustrates how supplementing the formal psychological assessment with more field-oriented tools can enhance the utility of the evaluation for the client and the psychologist. Of particular note is the client's inconsistency in performance that was evident in the naturalistic settings of home and work, but not seen in the formal psychological assessment. Inconsistency of performance is a common characteristic of individuals with neurological impairments, and can have a great impact on their ability to return to a job with or without modifications. Often individuals are able to perform the skills necessary for a given job, but have difficulty doing so consistently due to fatigue and their neurological condition.

It should be noted that impairment is defined by the ADA as involving major life activities of the person. Such activities include basic mobility and self-care skills for daily life, and basic cognitive skills for performing work and home activities. The individual's performance on a formal test may not be indicative of functional abilities or inabilities to perform home or work activities. As in the case above, the rehabilitation psychologist should obtain information about the person's abilities in everyday life, and seek to corroborate this information with the skills and deficits observed in the clinic and field assessment.

In writing reports on vocational findings, it is desirable to use functional descriptions rather than seeking to categorize and potentially stigmatize the individual by use of diagnosis. Moreover, such an approach is usually better understood by the employer considering the individual with the impairment for a job. If there is evidence of a particular problem, it should certainly be stated. The problem and its implications for the individual's ability to perform a job, however, should be described in functional terms as they relate to the workplace rather than relying on abstract jargon or categorization. For example, rather than simply stating the individual has a visual agnosia, it would be useful to also describe the individual's difficulty recognizing objects through vision. The individual may have difficulty with job tasks that are visual in nature. Such tasks might be better comprehended by the individual if they were simplified, if the task was explained verbally, or if there was an opportunity for hands-on experience with the task.

The psychologist must also make certain that the assessment process itself provides the individual with a fair opportunity to express his/her capabilities. One way that the psychologist can make the evaluation fair is by testing the limits of the individual's ability on a test. For example, the individual's score on a timed test could be obtained for purposes of comparing it with relevant norms. However, the individual might be given the opportunity to work beyond the time limit in order to see how effectively he/she works when there is a less restrictive time limit. This information can be useful in making suggestions for reasonable accommodation in the workplace.

Vocational Re-Entry

Having completed an assessment of the individual's cognitive and emotional status, the psychologist can then apply the information to a specific job or field in order to assist the individual with a job search

(Vandergroot, 1987). With respect to the job or workplace, a key feature of the ADA is the principle of reasonable accommodation. If the individual with a disability is unable to perform the job but is otherwise qualified, the employer must provide reasonable accommodation by making modifications in the job that enable the individual to perform the job or to engage in the usual activities in the workplace. The employer may avoid making such accommodations only if he/she is able to show that to do so would pose an undue hardship on the business. The individual with the impairment, however, must raise the issue of his/her need for the accommodation. If the matter is not raised, the employer is not obligated to make an accommodation.

The ADA states that the reasonable accommodation must be relevant to the disability and must be an effective means of enabling the individual with the disability to perform the job in question. The idea of reasonable accommodation is fairly straightforward when considering an individual with physical disabilities. A reasonable accommodation for an individual who uses a wheelchair for mobility would obviously include ramps and other modifications that allow that person access to the workplace, bathrooms, dining facilities, and every other aspect of the workplace that individuals who do not use wheelchairs can utilize. Individuals with neurological impairments pose a unique challenge to the determination of reasonable accommodation. To determine such clients' needs for accommodation the psychologist needs to perform a cognitive job analysis.

In such an analysis the psychologist analyzes the cognitive demands of the workplace. For example, an individual with an auditory-verbal memory problem might be unable to perform work duties because severe distractions that exist in the workplace interfere with his/her ability to attend to the stimuli in order to remember them. A reasonable accommodation might be to have that person perform the duties in a different area where distractions could be minimized or to provide a sound masking apparatus in the office. If the individual's problem is more specific to the actual encoding of auditory-verbal information, he or she might be able to perform work duties if he/she were given written instructions and visual illustrations about how to perform given work tasks.

Many of the ideas that are developed in cognitive rehabilitation programs can be applied in the workplace to fashion reasonable accommodations for the person with a traumatic brain injury. Table 5.1 lists some of the cognitive difficulties commonly noted in individuals with neurological impairments and some potential accommodations that could be made to a job. Clearly, such a generic list would need to be tailored to the specific job an individual was considering.

Unfortunately, the individual with severe neurological impairments usually does not have such discrete cognitive deficits. Because of this problem, rehabilitation professionals have utilized a job-coaching model to

Table 1. Examples of Cognitive Difficulties and Potential

Cognitive Difficulty	Workplace Accommodations
	Potential Accommodations
Reduces attention, distractibility	Enhancing signal stimuli through use of headphones, bold print, colors, or illustrations. Reduced distractions from noise by modifications in lighting, workplaces location, sound, and visual barriers.
Short-term memory impairment	Presentation and encoding of information in multiple modalities, such as instruction manuals that use verbal descriptors and illustration. Allowing employee to use memory cues or aids when performing task. Increasing opportunities for repetition and review of task.
Sequencing, planning	Numbering or color coding aspects of job to enhance sense of order. Providing visible models of completed work to aid in self-monitoring performance.
Visual spatial confusion	Simplifying diagrams for operation of machinery or completion of tasks. Using verbal cues or captions in diagrams. Providing written instructions to supplement visual instructions.
Verbal communication	Minimizing needs for verbal communication through nonverbal monitoring systems such as checklists. Supplementing written instructions or tasks with visual diagrams, illustrations or maps to enhance understanding.
Poor generalization of skills across situations	Increasing opportunities for repetition of tasks before switching tasks. Enhancing similarity in task components by performing tasks in same location or with same equipment.
Preservation, rigidity	Enhancing differences in task components by performing tasks in different parts of work space, using different styles or types of equipment for different tasks.
Fatigue, reduced speed	Reduce or avoid productivity requirements. Incorporate modifications in scheduling to allow for rests and review. Enhance sense of time passage through use of logs.

assist the person in return to work. In job-coaching, the individual is directly assisted in performing the work tasks by a coach who works side-by-side with the employee. The coach provides supplementary instruction, direction, and cueing on how to perform the job tasks. Ideally, the role of the coach diminishes with time as the employee becomes more independent on the job.

Job-coaching can be a reasonable accommodation if it is an effective means of helping the employee to perform the work, is relevant to the job and does not pose an undue hardship for the employer. Job-coaching and other accommodations made for individuals with cognitive and emotional difficulties should be monitored carefully and regularly (Hill, Cleveland, Pendleton, & Wehman, 1981). The job coach will provide some of this monitoring. In cases of more circumscribed modifications, the psychologist or employer may need to arrange a system for monitoring the accommodation to the client.

It is useful to brainstorm with the client about possible accommodations. Although the psychologist has assessment data regarding the client's abilities, the client is living with the particular neurological problems and may have some ideas about how the workplace could be modified to allow him/her to perform the job. It is also vitally important to include the employer in such discussions so that the job placement experience can be accomplished in a collaborative rather than antagonistic atmosphere.

The vocational placement of individuals with severe cognitive impairments who require daily supervision will often be directed by the psychologist or counselor from a vocational agency. Individuals with severe impairments may have limited ability to participate actively in the placement process. In such cases, the majority of the placement process may consist of the psychologist's contact and communication with a potential employer. Excellent model-supported employment programs for individuals with substantial cognitive impairments have been described (National Association of Rehabilitation Facilities [NARF], 1988; Pankowski & Rice, 1985; Wehman et al., 1988). In addition, resources such as the Targeted Jobs Tax Credit program and numerous organizations accustomed to identifying many cost-effective accommodations are listed in the ADA Technical Assistance Manual (EEOC, 1992). These resources are strongly recommended to those involved in vocational placement of clients with severe cognitive impairments.

Clients with only mild-to-moderate cognitive impairments, and individuals with physical limitations as the result of neurological impairments, are able to take a leading role in the job selection process. Many of these individuals are unable to find jobs because they lack job-seeking skills even though they may have the ability and qualifications to perform a given job. The rehabilitation psychologist can provide training in basic skills of interviewing, resume preparation and job hunting. This training can be expanded, in light of the ADA, to include information about clients' rights through ADA.

Ideally, the psychologist can assist such clients in preparing to apply for a position and be interviewed by the prospective employer. The psychologist can review test results with the client, and at the same time point out any behavioral observations about the client's motivation, work habits, and cognitive strengths that will be useful for the client to emphasize in a job-seeking situation. Knowing the general type of job being sought will help the psychologist and client focus their review of the client's potential. Possible accommodations relevant to client's needs can be discussed in advance, such things as alterations in the physical structure of the workplace, technical aids for using phones and computers, and safety needs, taking the client's capabilities into consideration should be discussed with the client so that he/she is able to discuss them confidently with the prospective employer. A list of resources to assist the employer could be prepared to present at the interview. The client's ability to present him/herself in a confident and responsible manner will minimize problems that may be encountered in obtaining employment.

Clients cannot, however, be expected to know the employer's level of awareness about the ADA, or the fears, attitudes, and experiences of employers they approach for a job, or one they return to following the onset of a disabling condition. In the event a client and potential employer cannot find answers to questions or solutions to problems on their own, input from the psychologist familiar with relevant issues may smooth the way to finding a resolution.

Case Example

S.J. is a 24-year-old woman with a college degree in English. She was seeking full-time employment as a technical writer in a corporate setting. During the last two summers in college she was an intern at United Cerebral Palsy and at a pharmaceutical firm. She had written public relations pieces and press releases in these positions. The position she now sought involved interpreting EPA regulations relevant to a new waste management company. An interview was scheduled by phone with the supervisor. The supervisor was stunned when S. J. arrived in an electric wheelchair, and was somewhat difficult to understand when she spoke.

S.J. has cerebral palsy and uses the wheelchair most of the time. Her articulation and vision are moderately impaired. Although she can maneuver her wheelchair, she has limited fine motor control. She requires occasional assistance in transferring from her chair to the toilet, but she cannot predict when she will need this assistance. She also requires some set-up for meals.

The beginning of the interview was handled awkwardly by the supervisor who apparently barely knew where to start. He made several complimentary comments about her portfolio. He asked her what sort of work she was seeking. After responding to this question, S. J. described how she goes about doing her work and the kinds of assistive devices she needs. She explained how she uses a voice synthesizer to read printed material and a tape recorder to dictate her writing. The interviewer then suggested that they tour the facility. During this tour, conversation was limited and the interview seemed to have come to a dead end. S. J. told the supervisor that it might be helpful for him to meet a psychologist at the university she knew who could serve as a resource to the company regarding workplace adjustments that would be needed to allow her to perform her job well. The supervisor agreed.

Prior to the meeting, S. J. and the psychologist planned their approach. S. J. would initiate and lead a discussion about her ability to manage the writing position. This strategy would demonstrate her knowledge and expertise regarding her abilities and the technical solutions for adapting to her physical limitations. In doing so, she would also demonstrate her personal competence and approachability. She would also be prepared to discuss some less obvious needs for accommodation to enable her to use toilet facilities and to manage meals on the job.

In the actual meeting, S. J. mentioned the increased ability of listeners to comprehend her speech over time. She added that she could handle personal computer use for limited periods of time. She then proceeded to discuss her toileting and mealtime needs. She proposed allowing her sister or another relative to join her at an early lunch hour for help with these activities. She also suggested posting a brief memo in the ladies room asking for volunteers to provide minimal personal care assistance (stand-pivot transfer) to a co-worker. These volunteers could be selected by interviews with S. J. and the personnel director. S. J. mentioned that she had used this system in college and the actual amount of time was less than 15 minutes per day.

The psychologist mentioned that some businesses qualified for tax credits for the costs of accommodations, in this case the cost of hiring an assistant for S. J. Also, recent advances in computerized voice synthesis might help S. J. on the job. The psychologist noted that S. J. might be eligible for purchase assistance for these items through an agency serving the visually impaired. Finally, the psychologist offered to provide future assistance as needed.

The meeting concluded with the supervisor stating that he felt that S.J. was a good candidate for the job and that she would be contacted after all other job candidates had been interviewed. About four weeks later S.J. was offered the job.

This example illustrates the importance of assisting clients in becoming aware of the employer's concerns in hiring someone with an impairment; particularly employers who have little experience with such situations. It is useful for clients to view the employer's concerns, at least initially, as the result of lack of information rather than a discriminatory attitude. By doing so, a positive problem-solving atmosphere can be fostered. Allowing clients to lead an open discussion of issues relevant to their disability opens the way for a discussion of possible work accommodations. In addition, by presenting a variety of ideas and options regarding accommodations, the client can display a number of personal qualities valued by employers.

When the psychologist presents useful ideas with an attitude of concern for the needs of both the employer and the employee, an ongoing problem-solving process of communication and information exchange can develop. The psychologist's knowledge of the wide variety of resources to assist the employer can foster an atmosphere of shared goals. The underlying goal of successful placement of the client in this positive atmosphere is more likely.

This example also illustrates the importance of considering the role of other employees in the workplace in accommodating the individual with an impairment. By participating in the accommodation of the worker with an impairment, other workers may feel more involved in the process leading to a greater degree of acceptance of the worker with an impairment.

On the Job

For the individual with neurological impairments who has received a commitment to be hired or is returning to a previously held position, the psychologist has a role in educating the employee about what to expect on the job and assisting in the design of reasonable accommodations.

The individual may face difficulties in adjusting to others' attitudes toward him/her. If the individual is returning to a job held prior to the injury, other employees may react with pleasure, caring, fear, confusion, embarrassment, anger, or solicitousness. The social stress caused by some of these reactions can disrupt the survivor's ability to manage the work situation and result in job failure. Education of the employee prior to taking the job may help him/her anticipate these reactions and handle them effectively.

Moreover, simply because other employees have a difficulty adjusting to the worker with a disability in the workplace does not justify isolating or otherwise restricting the activities and responsibilities of the worker with the disability. Situations have occurred in which employers, seeking to maintain peace in the workplace, have isolated the disabled worker from other employees. This action could constitute a violation of the ADA. The rehabilitation psychologist can take an active role in avoiding this situation by seeking to educate the employer and the other employees in the workplace about disability in general and, with the client's approval, about the specific needs of the client with a disability.

Some general counseling recommendations for work with individuals with neurological impairments are suggested by the ADA. Until the ADA, the individual with a disability had to see him/herself as limited and a potential burden to the employer. Only by the good graces of the employer and chance was the employee able to return to work. As a result, counseling interventions may have focused on helping the individual adjust to this role in the aftermath of disability.

With ADA, this interpretation of the client's role is unjustified. Rehabilitation psychologists must help the individual with a disability to see that he/she is entitled to and able to perform many of the same tasks as individuals without disabilities. Reasonable accommodation is not a special favor, it is the law. Psychologists must also help clients recognize their tendencies to engage in self-handicapping behaviors, putting themselves down, or seeing themselves as more disabled than is justified given their disability.

Case Example

M. H. is a supervisor in a state government office assigned to track returned overpayments in entitlement programs. A staff of seven report to her. She had held this position for 17 years when she was injured in a car accident. M. H. had an indeterminate period of loss of consciousness. She also had facial lacerations, fracture of the right orbit, and cervical and shoulder injuries. She was out of work for three weeks, but continued in physical therapy for a total of four months with minor adjustments to her work schedule until she was discharged from treatment.

Approximately one year after the accident M. H. began to complain about periods of "black outs," confusion, and problems with memory. A neuropsychological evaluation revealed deficits of efficiency of retrieval from long-term memory, distractibility, and reduced speed of processing. A neurologist diagnosed a seizure disorder. Follow-up discussions with M. H. revealed that she was having a number of problems on the job. She described her work station as cluttered, disorganized, and confusing. She reported having great difficulty finding her place if she were interrupted, as well as having problems deciding the order of tasks to be done. A treatment program that included individual psychotherapy, physical therapy, cognitive remediation, and participation in a support group was begun. She lost her driver's license as a result of the seizure diagnosis, and depended on friends for transportation to therapies and work.

After making these treatment plans, M. H. approached her supervisor to explain her need for some assistance in her work setting. She proposed that her psychotherapist come in weekly during the lunch hour. This request was approved. She received twelve therapy sessions at work.

During the first six months of her treatment, M. H. was easily able to make up for worktime missed while attending therapies because ample overtime work was available. Government cutbacks, however, suddenly eliminated all overtime. Workers were instructed to work only regularly scheduled hours except with special permission. When M. H. asked her supervisor for permission to continue making up time in early morning, evening, and Saturday hours she was refused. The supervisor stated that if he allowed her, he would have to make exceptions for everyone.

M. H. informed the psychologist that she would need to drop out of some therapies. The psychologist discussed the ADA guidelines with her, gave her some government brochures about the ADA, and encouraged her to discuss the material with her employer. She was reluctant to do so, fearing ill-defined future consequences if she pressed her case. Two weeks later she did present the materials and the supervisor said he would look into her request. After about one month during which M. H. had sporadic therapy attendance and no response from the employer, the psychologist proposed writing a letter on her behalf.

The letter, reviewed and approved by M. H., described the concept of reasonable accommodation. Flexible scheduling was specifically listed in the body of the ADA as an appropriate accommodation. The psychologist argued that flexible work schedules apparently continued to be permitted for certain circumstances at M. H.'s workplace, and her work would generally be completed on the same calendar date whether or not she attended therapies. Therefore, allowing a flexible schedule should not impose an undue hardship on the organization.

The supervisor was also referred to various resources including the ADA Technical Assistance Manual, and the state vocational rehabilitation office for further assistance. An accommodation was proposed that would allow M. H. to submit her therapy and work make-up schedules on a weekly basis. If any exceptional events or meetings should conflict with her proposed hours away, the situation would be discussed and negotiated. Finally, the psychologist proposed a meeting with the relevant parties and the psychologist if this proposal was unacceptable. The flexible schedule was approved two days after the supervisor received the letter.

This example illustrates the lack of familiarity, even in a government office, with the meaning of accommodation as encompassed by the ADA beyond the removal of physical barriers. In this example, the employee was not personally comfortable with her role of being her own forceful advocate. Perhaps this related to her level of cognitive impairment or to some other aspect of her personality. In any case, the psychologist made the decision to try to create change. While providing the relevant supervisor with resources, the psychologist also made very clear his/her intention to take a stronger advocacy role if necessary to assist the client.

Conclusion

Several other issues are worthy of mention but cannot be fully addressed within the scope of this paper. One, individuals of ethnic, religious, or sexual minorities who have disabilities may experience additional difficulties in their integration into the workplace. The rehabilitation psychologist needs to show continued sensitivity to these issues as they affect vocational re-entry.

Two, family issues are important in rehabilitation treatment. The ADA states that an employer cannot discriminate against individuals who are caring for a disabled family member, or have some association with a person with a disability. Family counseling should consider the impact of this on the individual with the disability and the family member's ability to work.

Finally, the rehabilitation psychologist has an ethical obligation to work on prevention of disabilities as well as treatment of them. This intervention can involve education of employers and employees about safety in the workplace to minimize work injuries. The psychologist can also suggest modifications of company policy related to factors that have been found to be related to the incidence of neurological impairments. These factors include alcohol and drug use, firearm safety, and health insurance plans that pay for preventive healthcare.

The ADA provides a tremendous opportunity for individuals with neurological impairments to enter or re-enter the workforce. This chapter has outlined some of the issues that the rehabilitation psychologist should consider in assisting these individuals. We have emphasized that the rehabilitation psychologist's role goes beyond that of an expert in diagnostic assessment and psychotherapy. The psychologist has a role in educating individuals with impairment, employers, and other employees in the workplace regarding disability and the rights of the person with a disability. The psychologist must also be an advocate for the individual with a disability, helping that person to recognize and attain his/her potential in the workplace and in society.

Acknowledgments

The authors thank Susanne M. Bruyère for her editorial guidance and support, and Alan Goldberg for his helpful review of this paper.

References

Cook, J. V. (1992). Returning to work after traumatic head injury. In M. Rosenthal, E. R. Griffith, M. R. Bond, & J. D. Miller (Eds.), *Rehabilitation of the adult and child with traumatic brain injury, Second Edition* (pp. 493–505). Philadelphia: Davis.

Equal Employment Opportunity Commission (1992). *A technical assistance manual on the employment provisions (Title I) of the Americans with Disabilities Act.* Washington, DC: Author.

Equal Employment Opportunity Commission & Department of Justice (1991). *The Americans with Disabilities Act Handbook.* Washington, DC: Author.

Hill, J., Cleveland, P., Pendleton, P., & Wehman, P. (1981). *Strategies in the disability follow-up of moderately and severely handicapped competitively employed workers.* Richmond, VA: Virginia Commonwealth University.

National Association of Rehabilitation Facilities (1988). *Supported employment resource guide* (G008745415). Washington, DC: U. S. Department of Education.

Pankowski, J., & Rice, B. D. (Eds.). (1985). *Supported employment: Implications for rehabilitation services.* Hot Springs, AR: Arkansas Research and Training Center in Vocational Rehabilitation.

Vandergroot, D. (1987). Review of placement literature: Implications for research and practice. *Rehabilitation Counseling Bulletin, 30,* 243–262.

Wehman, P., Kreutzer, J., Wood, W., Morton, M. V., & Sherron, P. (1988). Supported work model for persons with traumatic brain injury: Toward job placement and retention. *Rehabilitation Counseling Bulletin, 31,* 298–312.

Yeas, M. A. (1991). Trends in the incidence and prevalence of work disability. In S. Thompson-Hoffman, & I. Fitzgerald Stork (Eds.). *Disability in the United States: A portrait from national data* (pp. 161–183). New York: Springer Publishing Company.

·6·

Reasonable Accommodations in the Workplace for Individuals with Psychiatric Disabilities

Paul J. Carling

Introduction and Overview

With regard to the real integration of individuals with disabilities, American social policy and the behavior of American communities are both at a crossroads. On the one hand, sweeping new legislation establishes as a national goal the full integration of all people with disabilities into America's housing, workplaces, and community activities. On the other hand, the current reality of living with a disability most typically involves poverty, unemployment, inadequate or inappropriate housing, and particularly in the case of psychiatric (i.e. serious and persistent mental illnesses) or developmental disabilities, segregation. Another aspect of this paradox is the fact that mental health and vocational rehabilitation service systems have had a very poor history of success in achieving positive employment outcomes. Since these service systems themselves, until recently, have tended to discriminate against people with psychiatric disabilities in hiring, only a limited number of professionals have extensive experience with employing people with psychiatric disabilities, and in providing reasonable accommodations that will promote their success in the workplace.

In spite of this lack of history, both policy and practice in the mental health and rehabilitation fields are emphasizing mainstream employment in integrated settings, and employment of people with psychiatric disabilities, both within these fields as well as in the larger business community, is increasing. Similarly, there is a growing body of information about the nature of relevant reasonable accommodations for people with a variety of mental disabilities. The sweeping provisions of the Americans with Disabilities Act (ADA) are expected to reduce discriminatory barriers, accelerate hiring, and thus expand our knowledge of accommodations. Psychologists have valuable roles to play, both in assisting employers to design accommodations, and in assisting people with psychiatric disabilities to secure and maintain employment. Employers also have a critical need for relevant information in both the hiring context and that of ongoing employment. Longstanding employees may develop a serious mental illness, and, as will be described below, serious mental illnesses are defined relatively broadly in the law. An understanding of the larger context of the employment of people with psychiatric disabilities, and the changing nature of services that promote employment for individuals with this disability, will assist both psychologists and employers to understand how best to meet their obligations to persons with psychiatric disabilities, as required by the ADA.

Employment and Psychiatric Disability

Work is a fundamental aspect of life in America and as such, it pervades our cultural values. Americans below the age of retirement who do not work live apart from the mainstream of life in this country. Work has obvious economic benefits, and while we value "contributing members of society" (i.e. people who work), we also have a tradition of ambivalent social policy towards our citizens who do not work. On the one hand, we appreciate the importance of a social policy that provides a "safety net" for those who have disabilities and are unable to work, or those who become unemployed because of larger economic forces. On the other hand, that very "safety net" barely keeps pace with the cost of living. For instance, the federal income support program used by many individuals with psychiatric disabilities, Supplemental Security Income (SSI), even with state supplementary payments, currently provides a level of income that is not even adequate to rent "affordable" housing (using the federal definition of rent and utilities not exceeding 30% of one's income) in any county or metropolitan area of the United States (McCabe, Edgar, King, Ross, Mancuso & Emery, 1991). Nationally, the income of individuals with psychiatric disabilities is about $5,000.00 per year, typically placing these citizens within the "very low" income category, at twenty percent of median income or less. (Anthony & Blanch, 1987).

The impact of poverty on people with long-term mental illnesses is great, and increasingly there is research which shows that people's economic status is a better predictor of successful tenure in the community than are psychiatric symptoms (Lewis et al., 1988). People with psychiatric disabilities, who during an earlier time were "housed" in institutions, now primarily live in our communities (Goldman, Gatozzi, & Taube, 1981) and compete with the general public for such scarce resources as affordable housing and jobs. Increasingly, community mental health service providers are finding themselves attending to peoples' basic needs for food, shelter, and clothing, and there is a growing realization that the failure to meet these needs renders most clinical and rehabilitative interventions ineffective. Consequently, rehabilitation and mental health systems are searching for ways to enhance the economic status of people with psychiatric disabilities, and employment is one of the major strategies being explored. In this context, professionals are also coming to understand that people with psychiatric disabilities need a broad range of jobs, including very high level ones, and need room for career aspirations similar to those of all citizens.

Besides the obvious economic benefit, employment offers other important psychological and social opportunities. Work is often a major source of identity and self-esteem. Its participatory and public nature makes working one of the major ways that we experience social contact and a sense of belonging in society and in our community. As such, work can be a major vehicle for community integration, and unemployment excludes people with psychiatric disabilities from this common experience familiar to most Americans.

Despite the benefits of employment, both economic and psychological, employment rates for people with all types of disabilities remain very low in America. A Louis Harris (1986) poll recently concluded, in fact, that:

> "Not working is perhaps the truest definition of what it means to be disabled in this country. No other demographic group [than people with disabilities] under 65 of any size has such a small proportion of people working. Young blacks, for example, a group often singled out because of their very high level of unemployment, are much more likely to be working than are disabled Americans."

In addition, some research indicates that few of those eligible for vocational rehabilitation services actually receive them. The same Louis Harris (1986) poll of 1,000 individuals with all types of disabilities, found that while 60% of respondents were familiar with vocational rehabilitation services, only 13% had used them. Work remains a high priority for people with disabilities: 66% of respondents below the age of 65 who do not work, report that they want to work.

Mental health and vocational rehabilitation systems have a poor record of helping people with psychiatric disabilities to find, get and keep jobs, particularly jobs other than entry level ones. A study in Cuyahoga County, Ohio, for example, which followed 550 psychiatric patients from two state hospitals into the community to assess the services they received and the services they identified as wanting, found that only one in five received vocational services after discharge, although they were almost all unemployed. At the same time, 62% of those patients interviewed identified vocational assistance as a high need area, and 61% reported that their job placement needs were unmet. In addition, the study found that people very much wanted to work (Ohio Department of Mental Health, 1983). These findings indicate a failure on the part of both the mental health and the vocational rehabilitation service systems to provide support and opportunities for working.

A number of specific barriers to employment for people with all types of disabilities have been noted in the literature. The most frequently cited barriers to working according to the Harris (1986) poll were fear of loss of government health insurance (not disability benefits), employer attitudes (65% said that employers don't believe that they are capable of doing a job because of their disability), lack of education and skills, and transportation problems. As far as people with psychiatric disabilities are concerned, major barriers are the attitudes of vocational rehabilitation staff that these persons are the "last frontier" of clients (Ruffner, 1986), and the hardest to place in jobs (Wehman, Kregel & Barcus, 1985; Collington, Noble, & Toms-Barker, 1987). Fraser and Shrey (1986) reported on a study of vocational rehabilitation in agencies in the Northeast United States, and found that the most frequently occurring employment barriers were: vocational counselors' own personal misconceptions about mental illness (85%); negative attitudes among employers (81%); lack of accessible transportation (79%); economic disincentives (68%); large caseloads (65%); overall slowness of the rehabilitation process (62%); architectural barriers relevant to people with mental illness (58%); high unemployment rate nationwide (56%); difficulty in matching people to jobs (48%); client selection priorities within their own agency (44%); and too little time spent educating employers (40%). They conclude that these barriers are primarily manifestations of stereotypes, and a lack of training, knowledge, and experience among the job placement staff.

Employer attitudes toward mental illness are also a major problem. Parent and Everson (1986), in a comprehensive review of studies in this area, conclude that negative employer attitudes and their lack of knowledge about people with this disability accounted for most of the problems cited by employers for not hiring members of this group. Combs and Omvig (1986), echoing the findings of several other studies, found that employers generally do not believe that people with psychiatric disabilities are capable of working and, in ranking sixteen severe disabilities for relative employability, mental illness is ranked thirteenth. Finally, it is important to note that stigma against people with psychiatric disabilities is greater than for any other disability group (Anthony & Blanch, 1987).

There is a dearth of systematic information on actual employment rates for people with psychiatric disabilities. Various studies over the last fifteen years show a continuing pattern of very low employment. These studies, for example, indicate that about ten to twenty percent of individuals discharged from psychiatric hospitals obtain some form of employment (temporary, part-time or full-time) within two years; however, typical hospital recidivism rates range from fifty one to seventy five percent within two years, indicating a pervasive lack of ongoing community support (Anthony, Cohen, & Vitalo, 1978). Thus, "at the time of hospital discharge a person who is severely psychiatrically disabled has a much better probability of returning to the hospital than of returning to work" (Anthony & Blanch, 1987). A 1988 study of people with psychiatric disabilities in Vermont, conducted by the Center for Community Change through Housing and Support, reported an employment rate of 19% (Tanzman & Yoe, 1990) and a 1989 study, also conducted by the Center, consisting of interviews with inpatients at Vermont State Hospital, found that in spite of a relatively high unemployment rate, fewer than 40% of the interviewed patients had used vocational services in the year before their hospital admission (Tanzman, Wilson, King, & Voss, 1990). Similarly, recent data from a national evaluation study of five service demonstration projects in Washington, Rhode Island, Ohio, Wisconsin and Oregon, conducted by the Center, report an employment rate of 16%, of which less than 5% is in any kind of competitive employment. It is important to note that the individuals in these programs are living in the community and are receiving extensive support services (Livingston, 1990). In short, typically fewer than 20% of United States citizens with psychiatric disabilities are employed. Moreover, it appears that these rates have not changed substantially in the last decade (National Institute on Handicapped Research, 1979).

While the benefits of employment are fairly obvious, less is known about the effects of long-term unemployment. Research on unemployment has found that while the impact of joblessness on individuals is not uniform, it is apparent that prolonged unemployment is associated with increased rates of hospital admissions for psychiatric treatment, suicide rates and deaths from cardiovascular and alcohol related diseases. In addition, unemployment is associated with low self-esteem and stress, particularly if it is for extended periods (Liem & Rayman, 1982).

Undoubtedly, the disability benefit system has encouraged policy makers and service providers to think of people with long-term mental illnesses in terms of disability and not ability. The SSI benefit is provided based on an individual's impairment, and there are substantial economic disincentives for working full-time or even part-time built into the structure of the benefit. It may be true that we have, in fact, institutionalized low expectations about the capabilities of people with psychiatric disabilities.

The combination of the economic, psychological and social benefits of working, the risks associated with prolonged unemployment, and the low employment rates of people with psychiatric disabilities call for an examination of our vocational interventions, and, more fundamentally, our expectations about people with this disability. What we are doing does not seem to be very effective, and it is quite possible that these low employment rates are as much a reflection of ineffective services as they are of the course and nature of long-term mental illnesses.

Traditional Service Approaches Related to Employment

The reasons for such high unemployment rates among people with psychiatric disabilities then, are obviously complex (Carling, 1990), involving attitudinal, societal, policy, programmatic and personal barriers, as well as the status of the economy. At a societal and policy level, until recently, the fields of mental health and vocational rehabilitation proceeded from an assumption that people with severe and persistent mental illnesses were typically incapable of work. Thus, there were few, if any, mainstream or integrated employment opportunities made available in these systems, and, in fact, people with psychiatric disabilities were afforded few opportunities to provide input into policies, or into the design of vocational services. Pervasive discrimination, both in the community at large, as well as within mental health and vocational rehabilitation programs, resulted in most employment opportunities being closed off.

At a programmatic level, service models emphasized sheltered approaches or day treatment. Few staff were skilled or available for job development, for providing supports on the job, or for vocational or employment-related skills teaching needed to retain employment. Similarly, there has been a significant absence of resources, such as mainstream or integrated training and career development opportunities, that prepare people for meaningful work on a long-term basis. Traditional approaches to vocational rehabilitation for people with psychiatric disabilities have typically been transitional in nature. They are organized to help people "transition" into competitive employment (Knoedler, 1979) and are consequently time-limited. Generally, those individuals who do not achieve competitive employment through "transitioning" are relegated to day programs which do not provide employment-oriented services. In addition, these approaches implicitly assumed that there were just two kinds of permanent employment, competitive employment or sheltered workshops, and that some people would never be able to work in competitive settings (Anthony & Blanch, 1987). Within vocational rehabilitation programs, eligibility for services was typically linked to potential success in competitive work settings after a relatively short period of training, an approach which often excluded the great majority of people with psychiatric disabilities.

Lack of knowledge appears to have played a major part in narrowing the possibilities for employment. There is a paucity of published literature, for example, on the preferences and desires of people with psychiatric disabilities for work, or about the meaning of work in their lives. Similarly, unlike the case with other disability groups, until recently, there has been virtually no systematic information available to those who would promote employment opportunities, such as employers, service providers and advocates, about the specific supports people need on the job, and the alterations that can be successfully made in employment settings, work routines or specific job descriptions that would make it more likely for a person with a psychiatric disability to succeed in the workplace. To be sure, readers of such specialized and highly useful journals as *Psychosocial Rehabilitation Journal* or *Innovations & Research in Clinical Studies, Community Support and Rehabilitation* (both available from Boston University's Center for Psychiatric Rehabilitation) have access to such information, but these are not routinely used by most employers, service providers or advocates.

Emerging Policy Trends

Fortunately, we are witnessing broad changes with regard to policies, programs and advocacy that hold the promise of enhanced integration in general for people with psychiatric disabilities (Carling, 1990), and for expanded employment options as well (Wilson, Mahler, & Tanzman, 1991). At a national policy level, landmark legislation such as the Fair Housing Act Amendments and, most specifically, the Americans with Disabilities Act (ADA), prohibits discrimination based on disability.

At the same time, major policy changes in mental health and rehabilitation systems are underway nationally which emphasize the empowerment and full participation of people with psychiatric disabilities and their families in policy and program development, and which promote the goal of mainstream or integrated employment opportunities, both full-time and part-time. This "paradigm shift" (Ridgway & Zipple, 1990; Carling, 1990) emphasizes the changing view of people with psychiatric disabilities from patients, or service recipients/consumers, to full community members, with the same rights to integrated housing, work and social networks as all other citizens. Two policy statements recently enacted by the National Association of State Mental Health Program Directors (NASMHPD, 1989; NASMHPD, 1990) are illustrative of this shift.

*NASMHPD Position Paper on Consumer Contributions
to Mental Health Service Delivery Systems (1989)*

"The National Association of State Mental Health Program Directors (NASMHPD) recognizes that former mental patients/mental health consumers have a unique contribution to make to the improvement of the quality of mental health services in many areas of the service delivery system. The significance of their unique contributions stems from expertise they have gained as recipients of mental health services, in addition to whatever formal education and credentials they may have.

Their contribution should be valued and sought in areas of program development, policy formation, program evaluation, quality assurance, system designs, education of mental health service providers, and the provision of direct services (as employees of the provider system). Therefore, ex-patients/consumers should be included in meaningful numbers in all of these activities. In order to maximize their potential contributions, their involvement should be supported in ways that promote dignity, respect, acceptance, integration, and choice. Support provided should include whatever financial, educational, or social assistance is required to enable their participation.

Additionally, client-operated self-help and mutual support services should be available in each locality as alternatives and adjuncts to existing mental health service delivery systems. State financial support should be provided to ensure their viability and independence."

*NASMHPD Position Statement on the Employment of
Persons with Severe Psychiatric Disabilities (1990)*

The National Association of State Mental Health Program Directors (NASMHPD) recognizes the fundamental importance of integrated, paid, and meaningful employment to the quality of life for persons with severe psychiatric disabilities. Chronic unemployment can lead to isolation, poverty, and despair in any adult, and the current high rate of unemployment among people with severe psychiatric disabilities—estimated at 85% or more—must be lowered. This lack of jobs is a major barrier to successful community living, a personal loss to people who wish to work, and a societal loss to employers and taxpayers who would benefit from their inclusion in the workforce. State mental health authorities should assume a leadership role in significantly increasing the rate of employment among individuals with psychiatric disabilities.

Employment support must be an integral component of comprehensive community support programs. State mental health agencies should cooperate with consumers, family members, mental health professionals, private businesses, taxpayer groups, and other advocates to: focus existing public and private resources (such as the state/federal vocational rehabilitation program and state services for unemployed citizens) to better serve persons with psychiatric disabilities; expand supported employment opportunities; re-direct public funds away from segregated day programs and toward community-based employment programs; and reduce the disincentives still present in SSI and SSDI policies for recipients returning to work. Employers must be educated about the potential of persons with psychiatric disabilities to become valued workers.

NASMHPD supports the goals of the Americans with Disabilities Act of 1990: to eliminate unfair treatment of and discrimination against qualified workers with disabilities, improve access to mainstream resources, and to mandate the assessment of disabled applicants' qualifications with consideration of accommodations and support services. We acknowledge employment as an important route to economic empowerment and independence for consumers of mental health services. We will work to increase their opportunities to become productive members of American society."

Much of this evolution of policy has been facilitated by federal legislation, in particular, the Rehabilitation Act Amendments of 1986, (PL 99-506). This bill provided for the delivery of supported employment to many individuals who had not been previously eligible for vocational rehabilitation services, and specified criteria for the provision of these services. The 1992 reauthorization of the Rehabilitation Act modifies supported employment rules to make them more appropriate to psychiatric disabilities, and places major emphasis on choice, integration, and successful implementation of the Americans with Disabilities Act. A key element of the Rehabilitation Act Amendments of 1992 is a presumption that people with severe disabilities can benefit from vocational rehabilitation services to obtain gainful employment outcomes. This replaces the previous standard which assessed people for eligibility for services based on a judgment about the feasibility of their eventual employment, a standard that has historically been used to screen large numbers of people with psychiatric disabilities out of vocational rehabilitation services.

Emerging Practice Trends

Historically, vocational services for people with psychiatric disabilities have employed a variety of program "models," including sheltered workshops and transitional employment. Between 1983 and the present, there has been a proliferation of research on strategies for placing, training and supporting individuals with mental retardation in mainstream employment (Gifford, Rusch, Martin & White, 1984; Wacker, Berg, Berrie & Swatta, 1985; Lagomarcino & Rusch, 1988). Subsequent to the research related to individuals with mental retardation, research on strategies for supporting individuals who are mentally ill (psychiatrically disabled) began to emerge in the literature (Anthony & Blanch, 1987). As a result of these and other earlier studies (General Accounting Office, 1980; Greenleigh Associates, 1975; U.S. Department of Labor, 1977; 1979; Whitehead, 1981) regarding the poor vocational outcomes associated with day treatment, day activity and sheltered workshop models, new models began to emerge during the 1980s which were based on the notion that individuals with disabilities should have access to paid employment in integrated community settings. This change in focus is a result, in part, of the shift in the overall design and delivery of mental health service systems from residential mental hospitals to a community support systems model which goes beyond symptom reduction to rehabilitation and the provision of supports essential for re-integration into the community (Turner & TenHoor, 1979; Stroul, 1989). Trends within the fields of mental health and vocational rehabilitation which are likely to affect employment levels include the widespread adoption of a psychiatric/psychosocial rehabilitation approach (Anthony, 1990), and a growing acceptance of supported employment as the major focus of program development.

In recent years, drawing from advocacy work on behalf of individuals with mental retardation, mental health in the 1980s has shifted its approach to vocational rehabilitation towards employment in mainstream work settings. The central strategy used to promote success in integrated settings is the supported employment approach. This approach attempts to address a problem inherent in transitional employment and sheltered workshop approaches, which had focused on preparing people for competitive jobs which never seemed to develop. The supported employment approach departs from the "train and place" approach of transitional employment by first finding a job, and then providing the specific support and training necessary to help a particular individual perform successfully at the job. In addition, the supported employment approach is based on a philosophy that individuals with disabilities can do real work; the question is identifying and providing individuals with the appropriate assistance. The goal of supported employment is paid employment in competitive job settings for all people with disabilities.

Key aspects of this "paradigm shift" (Carling & Besio, 1992) include a change in focus: (1) from a continuum of vocational programs to an array of learning and work opportunities; (2) from vocational rehabilitation as therapy or treatment, to using work itself, and associated supports, to promote recovery; (3) from transitional approaches, to permanent or stable approaches; (4) from group "placements" in vocational "slots," to individual arrangements which people choose for themselves; (5) from a focus on using eligibility criteria, assessment, and training, and then placement, to offering employment and related supports to whomever wishes to work; (6) from requirements that people continue to receive services as a condition of keeping their jobs, to a focus on regular employer/employee relationships and benefits; and (7) from a pattern in which mental health's and vocational rehabilitation's roles were central as program operators, client sponsors, and funders, to a different set of roles as linker, broker, case manager, and provider of ongoing support.

What then are the characteristics of effective work assistance? Carling and Besio (1992) have identified the following common components of successful approaches to employment for people with psychiatric disabilities:

Approaches focused on Career Planning

- Identification of vocational goals
- Skills and interests identification
- Environmental needs assessment
- Resume development

Approaches focused on Job Access

- Identification of potential jobs
- Training in job interview skills
- Assistance with arranging interviews
- Assistance with clothing and transportation
- Identification of references

Approaches focused on Job Retention

- Assistance with "learning the ropes"
- Clarification of job expectations
- Emotional assistance
- Skills training assistance
- Support to employer and other staff, including on-call assistance, and identification of reasonable accommodations
- Facilitate Peer Support Opportunities, On-Site and Off-Site
- Provide Services and Benefits Coordination
- Assure Confidentiality

Hiring People with Psychiatric Disabilities as Service Providers

Each of these trends in policy development and program models has increased interest in hiring people with psychiatric disabilities, both within mental health and rehabilitation agencies, as well as in the larger workforce in the community. There are a number of indications that this interest in directly hiring individuals is at least occurring within mental health agencies. A recent NIDRR-funded national survey of mental health programs offering housing and community supports, conducted by the Center for Community Change through Housing and Support (Yoe, Carling & Smith, 1991), found that programs that are emphasizing the new integration paradigm are more likely to hire people with psychiatric disabilities in a wide range of positions. The experience base of these programs is a valuable one. In a national survey of consumer roles in housing and community support programs, conducted by the Center, significant challenges and benefits were identified by the 93 agencies that had hired people with psychiatric disabilities (Wilson, Mahler & Tanzman, 1991). The benefits, according to respondents, far outweighed the challenges. These findings are summarized below:

Challenges for the Consumer Staff

- Reduced public benefits
- Relationships with other clients may change
- Need to continue to address own needs, symptoms
- May be especially sensitive to job stress
- Difficulties in taking on new staff role
- Stigmatization, distrust from other peer staff

Challenges for the Organization

- Over-involvement by organization
- Confidentiality issues
- Comraderie may interfere with clinical decisions
- Have high expectations for clients, lack patience
- Poor clinical skills, self-disclosure
- Need more training time than other staff
- Need more supervision than other staff
- Symptoms may interfere with performance

- Absenteeism due to illness
- Inconsistent reliability
- Rehospitalization leaves staff shortages
- Turnover rate
- Higher costs of health insurance
- May not have meaningful work for highly skilled consumer advocates
- Need to spend time educating staff about benefits, process
- Process of having consumer staff takes time

Benefits Related to Personal Attributes of the Consumer Staff

- Personal knowledge of mental illness
- Better understanding of clients' needs/issues
- Empathy, sensitivity, compassion
- Less professional "ego" to distance them from clients
- Clients relate better to them
- More able to deal with bizarre symptoms
- Better understanding of medication issues/side effects
- Highly motivated, dedicated, committed to the job
- Willing to exceed what is expected
- Dependable
- Flexible in their work assignments
- Effective advocates for the system and for individuals
- Have good resources, contacts

Benefits to Consumer Staff

- Preserves dignity
- Personal growth, increased self-esteem, empowerment
- Provides job opportunities
- Increased income

Benefits to the Organization

- Enhances staff awareness of consumers' capabilities
- Provides valuable insight regarding good treatment strategies
- Increases staff sensitivity toward clients and their needs

- A source of constant education for staff without disabilities
- Gives the organization an informal perspective
- Provides consumer perspective/concerns to administration
- Programs, services are more relevant and attractive
- Provides quality control, "keeps us honest, on our toes"
- Increases organization's credibility with its clients
- Family and consumer groups are more supportive
- Good for the organization's image, good "public relations"
- Provides evidence of the organization's philosophy
- Well-performing employees
- Need less staff orientation time
- Helps with human resource shortages

Benefits to Clients

- Relate well, more directly to clients
- Role models for others
- Enriches services

Benefits to Society

- Effective, valid spokespeople for community education
- Decreases stigma, provides examples for the community

An important finding of this survey is that people with psychiatric disabilities are being hired in virtually all job categories and at all levels of these organizations, from senior management to entry level roles, from full-time to part-time positions, indicating both the range of positions that people can hold, as well as the potential variety of accommodations needed. As an example, a successful organization of ex-psychiatric patients, Mind Empowered, Inc. in Portland, Oregon, which began as a NIMH Community Support demonstration peer support project in 1988, was subsequently funded by the state to mount an intensive clinically oriented program to help a number of patients with a long history of institutionalization at a nearby state hospital, to return successfully to the community. The program organized itself into "continuous treatment teams," and began recruiting psychiatrists and planning how to "re-train" the psychiatrists they hired in a consumer self-help and empowerment approach. To their surprise, they found that several of the psychiatrists who applied reported that they too had a psychiatric disability, and were seeking employment in a setting where that was an asset, not something to be hidden (Smith, personal communication).

Reasonable Accommodation and Psychiatric Disabilities

In spite of this valuable information from the few available studies, it is clear that most change is occurring at a policy and program level, in the absence of easily accessible and specific information on those reasonable accommodations that are especially relevant to people with psychiatric disabilities. The fact that hiring is now taking place, even on a limited basis, is an extremely valuable opportunity to provide the field with systematic knowledge based on the actual experience of designing accommodations. The lack of availability of this information is a major impediment to further progress, since merely hiring, without a systematic approach to accommodation, may in fact lead to significant failure in the employment setting. Specifically, employers in the private sector, professionals who are offering employment in mental health and rehabilitation agencies, or who are assisting employers and individuals with a disability to create successful employment opportunities, and those who are seeking and/or advocating for such opportunities—people with a psychiatric disability, their families, other advocates—all have specific information needs that must be addressed.

Implications of The Americans with Disabilities Act

The ADA prohibits discrimination on the basis of disability in hiring and promotion. Further, employers must make "reasonable accommodations" to the disabilities of "qualified" applicants, unless doing so would impose an "undue hardship." "Qualified" means that, but for the disability, people can perform the essential functions of the job. "Undue hardship" is defined as "an action requiring significant difficulty or expense," and "reasonable accommodation" is defined as "any modification or adjustment to a job or the work environment that will enable a qualified applicant or employee with a disability to perform essential job functions" (U.S. Department of Justice, 1991). The disability must be known to the employer, and the individual must request an accommodation (U.S. Department of Justice, 1991). However, employers are not permitted to inquire about a disability prior to employment and an individual may choose not to reveal a prior psychiatric history at the time of hiring. If the person subsequently develops symptoms that require accommodations, the employer is obligated to respond. Similarly, a long-term employee with no previous psychiatric history may develop a serious mental illness and need accommodations to continue working. Thus, the accommodations that are discussed below are equally relevant to those persons whose psychiatric disability is or is not known at the time of hiring, as well as those employees who develop this disability after hiring.

It should be noted at the outset that, as with any sweeping new legislation, many of the provisions of the ADA have not been completely clarified, either through regulation or through the inevitable litigation that follows the enactment of major legislation. Parry (1993) provides a very useful, detailed, and current summary of both the ADA's ambiguities and evolving case law in this area.

In an excellent summary of the major provisions of the Act, the Mental Health Law Project (1992, p.2) points out that "it is now illegal for employers to:

- ask job applicants about psychiatric treatment—past or present;

- deny a job to someone with the necessary experience and skills because of the person's past or current psychiatric treatment or possible future treatment;

- deny a job or promotion because of a belief that a person with a mental disability won't be able to "handle" the job;

- refuse to make reasonable modifications in workplace rules, schedules, policies or procedures that would help a person with a mental disability perform the job;

- force an employee with mental disabilities to accept a workplace modification;

- contract with other organizations and individuals that discriminate against people with mental disabilities; or

- retaliate against people with mental disabilities for asserting their rights."

Each of these prohibitions has major implications for people with psychiatric disabilities. However, since the disability is often not obvious, and because of widespread stigma and discrimination, or simply as a statement of self-sufficiency, many individuals choose not to identify themselves as disabled. If they do self-identify, there is a major concern expressed by most authors in this area (e.g., Mancuso, 1990; Harp, 1991; Parrish, 1991; Belisle, 1990; Belisle, 1991) that employers and co-workers will interpret any work or personal difficulties the individual has, as related to that disability, especially if the worker has previously asked for an accommodation.

It is clear that a major effort is needed to provide accurate information about psychiatric disabilities to employers, so that they can make accommodations for people requesting them. Similarly, there is a need for a major educational effort targeted to people with psychiatric disabilities, which assists them in understanding and exercising their rights. The ADA is particularly relevant to those persons with psychiatric disabilities who are seeking, or desire assistance in securing competitive employment positions (Haimowitz, 1991). Fortunately, in the months since the passage of ADA, some materials have been developed which inform people with psychiatric disabilities about their rights (U.S. Department of Justice, 1991; National Mental Health Association, 1991; Mental Health Law Project, 1992), but to date there has been relatively little information about reasonable accommodations based on actual experience, with the exception of Parrish (1991), summarized below.

By far, the most helpful document produced to date on reasonable accommodations for people with psychiatric disabilities is the Mental Health Law Project's (1992) guidebook on the ADA, titled: *Mental Health Consumers in the Work Place: How the Americans with Disabilities Act Protects You Against Employment Discrimination.* This guidebook focuses on Title I of the Act, related to employment discrimination. The following information is drawn directly from the guidebook, which contains more detailed explanations of the provisions of the ADA, and the reader is encouraged to consult the full text of this very useful resource.

Who Is Covered By the ADA?

Title I applies to all private employers with 25 or more employees (and after 1994 to those with 15 or more employees). It prohibits discrimination against "qualified individuals with a disability" in all aspects of employment including hiring, promotion, discharge, training, compensation, and any other conditions of employment. The law applies to people who currently have a disability, who have a history of disability, or who are perceived as disabled, and includes both physical and mental disabilities. With few exceptions (see Jones, Ch. 8, p. 154) any psychiatric diagnosis listed in the American Psychiatric Association's *Diagnostic and Statistical Manual* (DSM) qualifies as an impairment, but the individual must also show that the impairment substantially limits the person in performing one or more "major life areas," such as self-care, learning, working, thinking, communicating, perceiving, or maintaining social relationships. Examples of such substantial limitations include an inability to maintain a schedule or come to work on time, or to get along with others. These limitations must also be present, not only in a particular job setting, but in a broad range of jobs. The ADA protects workers who improve with treatment, but who are likely to face continuing challenges because of their disability, even if they have no active symptoms. People with alcoholism are also protected—whether active or recovered—but only persons who are recovered from drug abuse are protected. Jones (Chapter 8) provides a detailed discussion of the ADA provisions related to alcohol and drug abuse. The ADA also protects people with a history of mental illness, people who are perceived as having a mental illness, and friends or relatives of people with disabilities, such as parents who might not be hired based on fear that they would miss work due to their child's disability.

Because persons with psychiatric disabilities are often impaired in the major life activity of working, the ADA's definition of a person who is eligible for protection puts people with psychiatric disabilities in something of a "catch-22" situation, in that they must also be "otherwise qualified" to do the work, with or without a reasonable accommodation (Parry, 1993). An employer faced with these seemingly conflicting criteria may well ask, "If this person is work impaired, why should I hire him/her?"

Privacy Issues

The ADA prohibits questions about medical or psychiatric history, and limits questions to those that will determine whether the applicant can do the job. A medical examination may be required, but only after a job offer is made, only if the examination is clearly job related, and only if all applicants for a position are required to undergo such an examination. Employers may tell supervisors or managers about the disability, if the employer believes that the disability makes the employee subject to any restrictions, or if accommodations are required.

Challenging Employment Discrimination

In order to challenge discrimination, an employee must show that he or she (1) is a qualified individual with a disability; and (2) can perform the essential functions of the job, with or without reasonable accommodations. Employers may not claim that persons can't perform essential functions merely because they have a disability, or because they may not be able to perform them in the future, presumably because of the disability.

Reasonable Accommodations

According to the ADA, an accommodation is any change in a particular workplace environment, or in the ways things are usually done, that make it possible for a person with a disability to perform a job. Accommodations must always be determined on an individual and a voluntary basis. In order to receive an accommodation, the employee must identify as having a disability and must request an accommodation. Beyond obvious accommodations, the ADA recommends that employers engage in discussion with the employee to identify the need for specific accommodations, the selection of which is ultimately up to the employer. Further litigation may be needed to clarify the limits of ADA protection in cases in which employers offer accommodations that the individual refuses, based on a belief that the particular accommodation will not ameliorate the situation (Parry, 1993).

An accommodation is only required if it does not present an "undue hardship" to the employer, for example, if it is too difficult to arrange, or too disruptive to the workplace (Parry, 1993). The employer may also refuse to provide an accommodation if it will be too expensive, but is obligated to consider any outside funding that is available. Employees are not required to accept any accommodations, and employers may not require that a person participate in treatment. Employers cannot refuse to hire because of safety concerns, unless the employee poses a "direct threat," based on an objective specific individualized assessment.

Fear—based on stereotypes that all people with mental illnesses will engage in violent behavior—is an insufficient basis to fire, or fail to hire, a person with mental illness. Any assessment of a "direct threat" must be based on current medical knowledge and/or objective evidence that the person has recently committed overt acts of violence, or made threats which caused or directly threatened injury, and that such threats cannot be eliminated by reasonable accommodations. The Supreme Court (cited in Parry, 1993) notes that key factors to consider are duration of the risk, nature and severity of the potential harm, and the likelihood and imminence of the harm. In this connection, according to Parry (1993), one question receiving considerable attention, but as yet unresolved, is the extent to which an employer can require an employee with a mental impairment and a history of violence, to take a prescribed medication as a condition of employment.

Finally, an employer may not fire, punish or threaten a person who asserts their rights under the ADA. Complaints may be filed with the Equal Employment Opportunity Commission (EEOC), and may be further pursued in court. People with disabilities can secure help from various Legal Aid, Protection and Advocacy, and other support services to pursue such claims.

What are Reasonable Accommodations for People with Psychiatric Disabilities?

The lack of knowledge about what constitutes relevant accommodations for people with psychiatric disabilities may stem from several sources: the low level of experience of employers with this group; the very diverse and episodic nature of the variety of serious mental illnesses, and the unique characteristics of each; and the relatively low level of predictability as to how a specific disability will affect an individual's job performance. To complicate matters, the ADA states that individuals with disabilities are entitled to "auxiliary aids and services" that would allow them to participate in jobs or activities to the same extent as other people. Yet, specific examples of the aids and services relevant to persons with psychiatric disabilities are not delineated in the law or the regulations (Parry, 1993).

Harp (1991), an ex-patient and employer, focuses on those accommodations that may be made to the overall workplace, co-workers attitudes, specific benefits, and so forth, which are not reflective of the individual's actual disability, but result from society's stigmatized misunderstanding of psychiatric disability. For example, employers who hire people with psychiatric disabilities, yet fail to provide adequate mental health insurance coverage, are, in effect, operating an organization that may not be able to support these individuals in retaining their jobs. Harp, therefore, suggests that it is critical to see the organization and it's culture—not just the individual job—as a target of change; and stresses that, above all, employees with psychiatric histories must be viewed and treated in the same way as all other employees. To achieve this end, accommodations must be voluntary, discussed and consensual. He goes on to describe the importance of such specific accommodations as on-the-job peer counseling, altering job qualifications, liberal sick and leave policies, scheduling modifications, flexibility in assignments, modification of the work environment, flexibility in supervisory methods and, above all, patience, tolerance, and understanding. Finally, the essential nature of accommodations is that they must be individualized.

Harp (1991), like many others writing in this area, points out that these accommodations should be provided to all employees in an organization if the goal is to create healthy organizations. This echoes a clear conclusion of the mental health agencies hiring people with psychiatric disabilities, who reported (Wilson, Mahler & Tanzman, 1991) that the effect of hiring people with psychiatric disabilities was invariably to improve the level of individual attention and accommodation to all employees, and thus to create a more positive working environment. It is important to note that Harp's recommendations should be seen as a resource for proactive employers who wish to embrace the larger goals of the ADA, since many of these accommodations would not be required under the law.

Specific Challenges and Issues in Accommodation Within Mental Health and Rehabilitation Employment Settings

There are a number of specific contextual issues that present unique challenges when hiring people with psychiatric disabilities within mental health and rehabilitation organizations. These stem in part from the changing culture in these organizations, and from residual negative assumptions about the "differences" between people with and without a psychiatric disability, or about the employability of people with this disability (Belisle, 1990). As a result, changes are often required in the overall culture of these organizations if they are to become supportive of employees with psychiatric disabilities. These changes include: (1) recognition that current and former consumers are already employed in the work force—whether or not they have acknowledged their disability; (2) acknowledgement by these consumers of the role that receiving treatment has played in their level of skill at providing treatment; (3) encouragement of supervisors, researchers and others to cite their experience as consumers along with their other qualifications as experts; and (4) promotion of relevant and appropriately timed personal disclosure by staff at all levels of the organization (Belisle, 1990). Again, it should be noted that disclosure is not required by the ADA, and is always voluntary. On the other hand, if we are, in effect, to change the culture of our practice to value and welcome professionals who are also consumers, such disclosure becomes an asset for agencies, employees, co-workers, and clients.

Thus, reasonable accommodation within mental health and rehabilitation employment settings must be seen within the larger context of consumer empowerment and "voice" (Hyde, 1989). A number of effective strategies for increasing consumer "voice" in organizations have been identified (Curtis, 1990). These include: gathering systematic information about consumers' preferences for work and supports to guide the development of services; fostering meaningful participation on boards, advisory committees and other groups; development of self-help and mutual support activities; providing resources to help consumers organize; expanding decision-making about programs, rules, treatment, and personnel to people with disabilities; providing resources for public education by consumers, and developing peer-operated programs.

Examples of Specific Accommodations

Although there has been no systematic collection of comprehensive data about the types of "reasonable accommodations" which are most relevant to people with psychiatric disabilities, there is some information available, which is based on the experience of hiring and retaining workers with this disability. Parry (1993), in an analysis of the ADA's requirements, divides typical accommodations for people with mental disabilities into those needed at the time of hiring (e.g., change the time of the interview; change the interview surroundings; or change a pre-employment test), and those needed on the job (e.g., flexible scheduling; reasonable time off; restructuring jobs or duties; restructuring the work environment; sensitizing other employees; and job assistance).

The Mental Health Law Project's (1992, p. 19) guidebook provides a summary of specific examples, also drawn from the ADA itself:

- flexible scheduling, such as allowing an employee to take a certain number of hours off every week or to change working hours to accommodate visits to a therapist or clinic;

- providing extra unpaid leave for short-term medical or psychiatric treatment;

- offering an employee a private work space to eliminate the stress of working with large numbers of people, or arranging for an employee to work off-site, such as at home;

- restructuring job duties by changing when, or how, a task is accomplished, or switching assignments with another employee;

- providing job coaches or other individualized on-the-job-assistance;

- changing an employee's supervisor if another would be more patient and flexible; and

- educating co-workers to improve their attitudes toward people with disabilities.

Mancuso (1990) notes that relevant accommodations also include modified or part-time work schedules and relocation or modification of the physical setting to reduce environmental stimuli. The National Mental Health Association (1991) further adds reassignment of the employee to a vacant position if this would prevent the employee from being unemployed or the employer from losing a valuable employee" (p. 13). While illustrative, none of these examples move beyond some general definition of "psychiatric disability" to more specific and functional limitations that may require accommodation.

With regard to more specific accommodations that have been offered, The West Virginia University Job Accommodation Network (1991) has provided some examples of actual accommodations that have been made for people with psychiatric disabilities in response to such functional limitations as "mental stress," "disorientation when in a strange environment," "memory difficulties," "agoraphobia," "anxiety and stress in crowded areas," or "stress, anxiety and depression due to seasonal changes." Focusing on such specific functional issues allows the development of interpersonal and environmental modifications that are more reasonable and more likely to be effective. Mancuso (1990) also provides a number of specific examples of accommodations that have actually been provided. These include:

- changes in interpersonal communication, such as arranging for all work requests to be put in writing for a library assistant who becomes anxious and confused when given verbal instructions; training a supervisor to provide positive feedback along with criticisms of performance for an employee re-entering the work force who needs reassurance of his/her abilities after a long psychiatric hospitalization; allowing a worker who personalizes negative comments about his/her work performance to provide a self-appraisal before receiving feedback from a supervisor; and scheduling daily planning sessions with a co-worker at the start of each day to develop hourly goals for someone who functions best with added time structure;

- modifications to the physical environment, such as purchasing room dividers for a data entry operator who has difficulty maintaining concentration (and thus accuracy) in an open work area; arranging for an entry-level worker to have an enclosed office to reduce noise and interruptions that provoke disabling anxiety;

- job modification, such as arranging for someone who cannot drive or use public transportation to work at home; restructuring a receptionist job by eliminating lunchtime switchboard duty normally handled by someone in this position; exchanging problematic secondary tasks for part of another employee's job description; and

- schedule modification, such as allowing a worker with poor physical stamina to extend his/her schedule to allow for additional breaks or rest periods during the day; allowing a worker to shift his/her schedule by an hour-and-a half twice per month to attend psychotherapy appointments.

Finally, Parrish (1991) completed a survey of individuals with a psychiatric disability and employers who had hired them. Most respondents were providing peer and other support services through NIMH Community Support Program funded demonstration projects and self-help programs focusing on people with psychiatric disabilities. She reports on a large number of specific accommodations that people found helpful:

- emotional supports, such as offering peer support, having an advocate available, praise and positive reinforcement, taking time to listen, staying in contact during a hospitalization, identifying co-workers willing to provide support on the job, making employee assistance programs available, providing on-site crisis intervention, providing access to a hot line during non-work hours, access to low cost, competent clinical services, and allowing telephone calls for support during work hours;

- concrete supports, such as assistance with child care, assistance with disability and income support paperwork, rights and legal advice for addressing grievances;

- prevocational and transitional work assistance, such as help with resumes, interviewing, transportation, use of a job coach, and help to purchase clothing, providing counseling related to requesting accommodations, developing a volunteer schedule, and using internships;

- flexibility, such as liberal leave policies, backup coverage during extended leaves, allowing people to work at home, flexible hours and self-paced work load, part-time job options, job-sharing, and flexibility about changing jobs or supervisors, rather than leaving;

- effective supervision, such as honest and frank initial interviews focused on potential problems and strategies for handling them, up-front discussion of the disability, in-depth clear explanation of duties, clear and supportive supervision, including easy access to the supervisor, time set aside to discuss work goals and needs;

- adequate wages and benefits, health insurance without limitations on mental illness coverage, advocacy with insurers, and permitting sick leave for emotional problems;

- training and education, such as individualized training, as well as ongoing training;

- transportation, including providing subsidies, helping to obtain a driver's license, or providing insurance; and

- dealing with co-workers attitudes, including recognition of the unique strengths of people with psychiatric disabilities, open discussions with workers with and without disabilities, rewards for examples of support, and penalties for overt behaviors which impede the success of people with disabilities.

Based on this information, Parrish proposes a set of guidelines for providing reasonable accommodations "in a manner that does not stigmatize or disempower the individual" (p.4). These guidelines include: (1) an employer "mind set" of respect, that does not view the person as different, recognizes individual strengths and contributions, and is willing to engage in joint problem solving; (2) involving the person in decision making, including determining reasonable accommodations; (3) designing accommodations that are voluntary and that are unique to the individual, and being clear about what does and does not require an accommodation; (4) periodic updating of job descriptions and of accommodations; (5) development of a crisis or stress management plan; (6) respecting confidentiality, and assuring that disclosure will not adversely affect the individual; and (7) encouraging the use of supports, such as self-help, but not promoting continued use of on-site supports, such as a job coach—which some consider stigmatizing—longer than needed.

Parrish also reports on some of the specific difficulties that individuals with psychiatric disabilities and employers have encountered with regard to reasonable accommodation. These include:

- disclosure issues, such as reluctance to reveal one's history based on fear of not being hired, or being fired when problems surface;

- lack of assertiveness in requesting accommodations;

- confusion about what constitutes a "reasonable" accommodation, and what constitutes "preferential treatment;" distinguishing between "accommodating" and "permitting" dysfunctional behavior; balancing needs for supervision with the need for autonomy;

- resource problems, such as the lack of support services or back-up staff to do the job during absences; and high demand on supervisor's time and energy; and

- communication problems, such as negative, fearful, exclusionary behaviors among non-disabled staff; resentment by staff of the accommodations provided; lack of ongoing communication between employees and employer.

Each of these information sources, while not based on empirical research, can be very helpful to psychologists in working with employers and with individuals with psychiatric disabilities who are seeking employment. In conclusion, it is clear that while we have no empirical data on effective reasonable accommodations, there is already a great deal of information to assist employers, mental health and rehabilitation professionals, people with a psychiatric disability and their families, and other advocates, to expand access to employment, and to promote reasonable accommodations, based on the actual experience of hiring and retaining employees in a wide variety of work settings throughout the United States.

Helpful Roles for Psychologists

It is hoped that the material provided above will offer psychologists a broad range of tools to assist employers to meet their larger business goals, while promoting an inclusive workplace, in which people with a variety of disabilities can succeed. In this respect, the psychologist's role is a critical one, acting as a bridge between diverse interests. On the one hand, psychology's ethical standards promote integration of people with mental health problems, oppose employment discrimination, and position the practitioner as an advocate for full implementation of the ADA, rather than mere compliance. On the other hand, psychologists work with employers who are typically new to the hiring of people with psychiatric disabilities, and who may well be influenced by the very negative beliefs that have historically impeded integration. Employers are typically unaware of how these beliefs have prevented the individual with a disability from taking his or her rightful place as a fully participating citizen of the community, with all the rights and responsibilities accorded other citizens.

Working with People with Psychiatric Disabilities

Specific strategies for assisting the individual with a psychiatric disability include listening carefully for the person's goals and choices, and assisting the person to develop a viable plan for employment, including a plan for the supports the person will need both on and off the job site. Second, individuals often require assistance to develop and practice interpersonal and interview skills, including the ability to effectively present themselves, particularly after a long period of absence from work, and to explain any gaps in employment. Very importantly, people often need help in figuring out exactly how to represent and discuss the psychiatric disability itself.

Knowledge of the related employment provisions of the ADA is essential. It is also important, however, to stress that some people choose not to reveal their psychiatric disability to employers. That choice needs to be respected as legitimate, even if it carries with it the consequence of not allowing the individual to request specific accommodations at the time of hiring. Discrimination is an everyday reality in the lives of people with a history of mental illness, and we simply do not yet know enough to advise individuals on a particular strategy for dealing with such potential discrimination.

It appears to be the case that significant numbers of individuals with psychiatric disabilities may not need particular on-the-job accommodations. The availability of a strong support system outside of work helps in dealing with work-related problems, and may allow the person to choose not to disclose his or her psychiatric disability. Therefore, it is important for the psychologist to examine with the person the nature of his or her current support system, and ways that the support system can be mobilized to provide extra support during the transition into work. In some cases, after-hours employment support groups appear to be helpful, as is ongoing involvement with a self-help group. Individuals will also want to reexamine the quality of their connections with professional services at this point, and to develop a crisis plan, before any potential crises occur.

In some cases, the psychologist will serve as an advocate, or a case manager, prodding other service providers to offer access to needed supports. In other cases, the psychologist may serve as a referee, particularly when services or benefit programs, accustomed to dealing with individuals who are unemployed, insist on rigid appointment schedules, medication regimens, or other practices that may conflict with work requirements. Coordination of the work schedule with the medication regimen is especially critical, since dosages can either assist some individuals in the workplace, or greatly impede their work performance. Working itself represents such a major situational change that medication needs often change significantly during the transitional period.

In addition, the psychologist may be asked to serve as a communicator with the family. Not only must the individual who is working adapt to changes brought on by employment, but so must family members. Some family members may want guidance in how to be supportive to the individual during the transition to employment. In this context, it is important to note that anxiety is a common ingredient of change, and that anxiety can be higher in the context of a history of failed work attempts, both for the individual and the family.

It is also critical for psychologists to work closely with individuals in planning the financial transition from benefit programs such as Supplemental Security Income (SSI) or Social Security Disability Income (SSDI). In spite of recent reforms, these programs still contain serious work disincentives, most importantly, the termination of health care benefits through Medicare and Medicaid once a person is gainfully employed. (O'Keeffe (Chapter 1) discusses in more detail the issue of health insurance as it relates to persons with disabilities). In this regard, it is important to consider various jobs in light of the benefits they offer, and in light of contingency plans for health care coverage, in the event that a particular job does not work out. It is important for the psychologist and the individual to work closely with someone in the community who is very knowledgeable about these benefit issues. It is also very useful to work closely with vocational rehabilitation staff, since they have access to a number of specialized training programs, transitional funding, and other resources to assist in returning to work.

Finally, it is important to negotiate a clear set of expectations about whether and how the psychologist will be involved in the workplace. While some individuals will choose to keep such relationships completely separate, others may prefer that the psychologist assume a communication and negotiation role, perhaps directly with the employer, in the event of problems on the job. One risk is that the employer may, in such cases, focus excessively on the disability, since other workers do not typically initiate such arrangements. Any such interventions, of course, must be determined by the person, not by the psychologist. The watchwords here are flexibility, openness to the need for support, high expectations that the individual can succeed with minimal special supports, persistence in providing whatever supports are needed, continuous communication—particularly in the pre-employment and transition period and routinely afterwards—and a willingness to celebrate this significant accomplishment on the person's part.

Working with Employers

Psychologists face just as varied a set of roles and activities with employers. These may include educating the employer about the nature of psychiatric disabilities, and about their responsibilities to comply with the ADA, including the requirement to provide reasonable accommodations and the need to examine those practices which are prohibited under the law. In this context, it is imperative for the psychologists never to allow themselves to be placed in a position of assisting employers to "meet the letter of the law," while continuing to exclude people with disabilities. In fact, the most helpful role is to assist employers to embrace the law, and to implement it in the context of the spirit it represents.

Employers need help to refine their interviewing procedures and to examine their health care benefits, although the ADA's provisions regarding health insurance are inadequate to address the myriad problems in this area. Employers also need to write detailed job descriptions, carefully spelling out the essential tasks of the job, and the required qualifications. They may also need specific education about those reasonable accommodations which are most relevant to individuals with psychiatric disabilities, and help in developing strategies for respectfully negotiating accommodations with individuals.

How then does the psychologist gain the knowledge he or she needs in order to be of assistance to employers? The psychologist can use the information provided in this chapter and its referenced sources, and can gain experience through visiting organizations in the community that have actively hired people with psychiatric disabilities. For those who are in a position to do so, they can hire individuals with psychiatric disabilities. This personal experience as an employer will be most valuable when serving as a consultant to other employers. Other ongoing sources of information for the psychologist include local self-help groups, and mental health programs that are promoting employment opportunities. These organizations are also valuable sources of support for individuals, so building positive relationships with them is essential.

Employers also need assistance to keep their role as an employer separate from that of a "counselor," a problem often encountered in human service settings. Additionally they may need assistance in setting clear and consistent policies for performance and for appropriate behavior on the work site, and in developing and implementing effective strategies for coordination with service providers, to the extent that the individual with a disability desires this coordination. In this connection it is helpful for the psychologist to review personnel policies, supervisory practices, and any accommodation plans that are developed. Psychologists can help employers plan for any extra supervision that may be needed, for back-up coverage in the event of absences, for policies that respect both accountability and confidentiality, and for developing grievance mechanisms that will anticipate any problems before they become major disputes.

Since so many examples of "reasonable accommodations" are, in fact, simply examples of effective management and supervisory practices, it can be especially helpful for psychologists to assess the overall organizational climate, and to suggest practices that would benefit all employees, not just those with disabilities. In this context, psychologists can be helpful in educating other employees about the process of integrating people with disabilities into the workforce, and the applicability of the ADA's provisions to anyone with a significant disability. Psychologists can perform valuable roles in problem solving and in the mediation of conflicts should they arise. Psychologists can also be helpful in team building and promoting team work before and after the hiring of employees with disabilities.

Regardless of specific strategies that psychologists may use in working with employers and with individuals with psychiatric disabilities, the essential skills needed to fulfill such a challenging set of roles are those of integrity, open communication, and commitment to the shared interests of the several clients involved. The promise of such a role is the ability to promote a "win–win" situation, in which employers are able to attract otherwise qualified workers who also have a disability and to promote an integrated workplace in which people with psychiatric disabilities are able to take their rightful place.

References

Anthony, W. A. (1990). *The philosophy and practice of psychiatric rehabilitation*. Boston University: The Center for Psychiatric Rehabilitation.

Anthony, W. A., & Blanch, A. (1987). Supported employment for persons who are psychiatrically disabled: A historical and conceptual perspective. *Psychosocial Rehabilitation Journal, 11* (2), 5–23.

Anthony, W. A., Cohen, M., & Vitalo, R. (1978) The measurement of rehabilitation outcome. *Schizophrenia Bulletin, 4* (3), 365–381.

Belisle, K. (1990). *Reasonable action and affirmative accommodation.* Woonsocket, RI: Northern Rhode Island Community Mental Health Center.

Belisle, K. (1991). *Transformation and paradox: Critical human resource development issues.* Woonsocket, RI: Northern Rhode Island Community Mental Health Center.

Carling, P. J. (1990). Major mental illness, housing and supports: The promise of community integration. *American Psychologist, 45* (8), 969–975.

Carling, P. J. (1991). *Employment and reasonable accommodation for people with psychiatric disabilities.* Training workshop presented at Howard Mental Health Services. Burlington, VT: The Center for Community Change through Housing and Support.

Carling, P. J. & Besio, S. W. (1992). Community integration of people with psychiatric disabilities: A comprehensive approach. Burlington, VT: The Center for Community Change through Housing and Support.

Collignon, F.C., Noble, J., & Toms-Barker, L. (1987). Early lessons from the Marion County Demonstration in integrating vocational and mental health services. *Psychosocial Rehabilitation Journal, 11*(2).

Combs, I.H. & Omvig, C.P. (1986). Accommodation of disabled people into employment: Perceptions of employers. *Journal of Rehabilitation,* 42-45.

Cook, J.A., Jusko, R.A., Gorman, B., Mock, L., Rosenberg, H., Naylor, K.E., & Jonikas, J. (1989). *Thresholds Annual Report: Fiscal Year 1989.* Chicago: Thresholds Research Institute.

Curtis, L. C. (1990). *Strategies for increasing and supporting consumer involvement in mental health policy/planning, management, and services delivery.* Burlington, VT: The Center for Community Change through Housing and Support.

Fraser, R.T., & Shrey, D.E. (1986). Perceived barriers to job placements revisited: Toward practical solutions. *Journal of Rehabilitation,* 26-30.

General Accounting Office (1980). *Better reevaluations of handicapped persons in sheltered workshops could increase their opportunities for competitive employment.* Washington, D.C.: General Accounting Office.

Gifford, O.L., Rusch, F.R., Martin, J.E., & White, D.M. (1984). Autonomy and adaptability: A proposed technology of maintaining work behavior. In N. Ellis & N. Bray (Eds.), *International Review of Research in Mental Retardation,* NY: Academic Press, Vol. 12, 284–314.

Goldman, H.H., Gatozzi, A.A., & Taube, C.A. (1981) Defining and counting the chronically mentally ill. *Hospital & Community Psychiatry, 32* (1), 21-27.

Greenleigh Associates (1975). *The need of the sheltered workshop in the rehabilitation of the severely handicapped.* Report to the Department of Health, Education, and Welfare, Rehabilitation Services Administration, New York.

Haimowitz, S. (1991). Americans with Disabilities Act of 1990: Its significance for persons with mental illness. *Hospital and Community Psychiatry, 42* (1), 23-24.

Harp, H. T. (1991). *A crazy folk's guide to reasonable accommodation and psychiatric disability.* Oakland, CA: Independent Living Support Center.

Harris, Louis & Associates, Inc. (1986) Disabled Americans' self-perceptions: Bringing disabled americans into the mainstream. Washington, DC: Harris, Louis & Associates.

Hyde, P. (1988). Implementing consumer choice. In P. J. Carling & S. F. Wilson, (1988). *Strategies for state mental health directors in implementing supported housing.* Burlington, VT: The Center for Community Change through Housing and Support.

International Center for the Disabled (1986). *The ICD survey of disabled Americans: americans Into the mainstream,* New York: Author.

Knoedler, W. (1979). How the training in community living program helps patients work. *New Directions for Mental Health Services, 2,* 57–66.

Lagomarcino, T.R., & Rusch, F.R. (1988). Utilizing self-management procedures to teach independent performance. In T.R. Lagomarcino, C. Huch, & F.R. Rusch (Eds.), *Self-management: Facilitating employee independence in supported employment settings,* Champaign, IL: University of Illinois, Secondary Transition Intervention Effectiveness Institute, Vol. 4, 141–174.

Lewis, D.A., Riger, S., Rosenberg, H., Wagenaar, H., Lurigio, A.J., & Reed, S. (1988). *Worlds of the mentally ill: How deinstitutionalization works in the city.* Northwestern University: The Center for Urban Affairs and Policy Research.

Liem, R., & Rayman, P. (1982). Health and social costs of unemployment. *American Psychologist, 37* (10), 1116-1123.

Livingston, J. (1990). *National evaluation of five service demonstration projects.* Burlington, VT: The Center for Community Change through Housing and Support.

McCabe, S.S., Edgar, E.R., King, D.A., Ross, E.C., Mancuso, L.L. & Emery, B.D. (1991). *Holes in the housing safety net: Why SSI is not enough: A national comparison study of supplemental security income and HUD fair mar-*

ket rents. Burlington, VT: The Center for Community Change through Housing and Support.

Mancuso, L. (1990). Reasonable accommodations for workers with psychiatric disabilities. *Psychosocial Rehabilitation Journal, 14* (2), 15–16.

Mental Health Law Project (1992). *Mental health consumers in the workplace: How the Americans with Disabilities Act protects you against employment discrimination*. Washington, DC: Author

National Association of State Mental Health Program Directors (December, 1987). *Position statement on housing and support for people with long-term mental illness*. Alexandria, VA: NASMHPD.

National Association of state Mental Health Program Directors (December, 1989). *Position paper on consumer contributions to mental health service delivery systems*. Alexandria, VA: NASMHPD.

National Association of State Mental Health Program Directors (December, 1990). *Position statement on employment for persons with severe psychiatric disabilities*. Alexandria, VA: NASMHPD.

National Institute of Handicapped Research (1979). Past employment services aid mentally disabled clients. *Rehabilitation Brief, 30*, 1–4.

National Institute of Mental Health (September, 1987). *Guidelines for meeting the housing needs of people with psychiatric disabilities*. Rockville, MD: NIMH.

National Mental Health Association (1991). *Americans with Disabilities Act of 1990 (Public Law 101-336*. Legislative Summary Series. Arlington, VA: National Mental Health Association.

Ohio Department of Mental Health (1983). *A Symposium on community services to discharged psychiatric patients*. Columbus, OH: Ohio Department of Mental Health.

Parent, W.S., & Everson, J.M. (1986). Competencies of disabled workers in industry: A review of business literature. *Journal of Rehabilitation*, 16–23.

Parrish, J. (March, 1991). *Reasonable accommodations for people with psychiatric disabilities*. Informal Survey Report. Rockville, MD: National Institute of Mental Heath.

Parry, J.W. (1993). Mental disabilities under the ADA: A difficult path to follow. *Mental and Physical Disabilities Law Reporter*, 17(1), 100–112.

Ridgway, P. & Zipple, A. M. (1990). The paradigm shift in residential services: From the linear continuum to supported housing approaches. *Psychosocial Rehabilitation Journal, 13* (4), 11–31.

Roessler, R.T., Hinman, S., & Greenwood, R. (1985). *Enhancing employability through skill training and placement interventions.* Paper presented at the meeting of the International Association of Psychosocial Rehabilitation Services, Boston, MA.

Ruffner, R.H. (1986) The last frontier: Jobs and mentally ill persons. *Psychosocial Rehabilitation Journal, 9*, 35–42.

Simon, M. (1990). Making a difference: Ex-patients as staff. *Resources, 2* (1), 9–10.

Skelley, T.J. (1980). National developments in rehabilitation: A rehabilitation services perspective. *Rehabilitation Counseling Bulletin, 24*, 22–33.

Smith, G. (1991) Personal communication.

Stroul, B. (1989). Community support systems for people with long-term mental illness: a conceptual framework. *Psychosocial Rehabilitation Journal, 12* (3), 9–26.

Tanzman, B., Wilson, S., King, D., & Voss, W.J. (1990). *The Vermont state hospital cohort study.* A report to the Vermont Department of Mental Health. Burlington, VT: The Center for Community Change through Housing and Support.

Tanzman, B., & Yoe, J. (1989). *Vermont consumer housing and supports preference study* (Full Report). Burlington, VT: The Center for Community Change through Housing and Support.

Turner, J., & TenHoor, W. (1979). The NIMH community support program: Pilot approach to a needed social reform. *Schizophrenia Bulletin, 4*, 319–344.

United States Commission on Civil Rights (1983). *Attitudes toward the handicapped.* Washington, D.C., U.S. Government Printing Office.

United States Department of Justice (1991). *The Americans with Disabilities Act: Questions and answers.* Washington, DC: Civil Rights Division, U. S. Department of Justice.

United States Department of Labor (1979). *Study of handicapped clients in sheltered workshops, (VOL II).* Washington, D.C.: U.S. Department of Labor.

United States Department of Labor (1977). *Sheltered workshop study: A nationwide report on sheltered workshops and their employment of handicapped individuals, (Vol. I).* Washington, D.C.: U.S. Department of Labor.

Wacker, D.P., Berg, W.K., Berrie, P. & Swatta, P. (1985). Generalization and maintenance of complex skills by severely handicapped adolescents following picture prompt training. *Journal of Applied Behavior Analysis, 18* (4), 329–336.

Wehman, P., Kregel, J., & Barcus, J.M. (1985). From school to work: A vocational transition model for handicapped students. *Exceptional Children, 52*, 25–37.

West Virginia University Job Accommodation Network (January, 1991). Accommodations made/suggested for individuals with some type of mental impairment. Morgantown, WV: WVU / JAN.

Whitehead, C. (1981). *Final report: Training and employment services for handicapped individuals in sheltered workshops.* Washington, D.C.: Office of Social Services Policy, Office of the Assistant Secretary for Planning and Evaluation, U.S. Department of Health and Human Services.

Wieck, C. (1988). The transition to productive employment: Legal and policy issues. In B. Ludlow, A. Turnbull & R. Luckasson (Eds.), *Transitions to adult life for people with mental retardation: Principles and practices,* (pp. 215–231). Baltimore: Paul H. Brookes Publishing Co.

Wilson, S. F., Mahler, J., & Tanzman, B. (1991). *A technical assistance report on consumer and ex-patient roles in supported housing services.* Burlington, VT: The Center for Community Change through Housing and Support.

Yoe, J. T., Carling, P. J., & Smith, D. J. (1991). *A National survey of supported housing programs for persons with psychiatric disabilities.* Monograph Series on Housing and Rehabilitation in Mental Health. Burlington, VT: The Center for Community Change through Housing and Support.

· 7 ·

The Americans with Disabilities Act and Injured Workers

Implications for Rehabilitation Professionals and the Workers' Compensation System

Christopher G. Bell

The Americans with Disabilities Act (ADA) is landmark civil rights legislation; however, few lawmakers seemed to foresee the breadth and depth of its impact on business. Perhaps the least anticipated impact was its potential effect on workers' compensation. Despite many newspaper accounts projecting catastrophe, there is not a single line in the ADA even mentioning workers' compensation. There was never any doubt that injured workers could be "individuals with disabilities" protected by the ADA; nonetheless, at the time the legislation was being crafted (during 11 congressional hearings and five committee markup sessions), virtually no attention was paid to its overlapping jurisdiction with workers' compensation.

How could this have happened? One explanation is that people in the disability rights community who lobbied for the ADA had no knowledge of workers' compensation. They viewed civil rights and benefits for persons with disabilities as apples and oranges; two distinct and separate approaches. After the first six months of ADA employment discrimination charges filed with the Equal Employment Opportunity Commission (EEOC), it appears that injured workers will be the principal beneficiaries of the ADA; 4,324 ADA charges had been received by January 31, 1993. Over 80 percent of the charges are from current employees rather than applicants. "Back impairment" is the largest single disability category (16.8 percent) and 40 percent of the bad back charges were discharge claims. While little is known about the details of the specific charges, because the ADA requires the EEOC to keep such information confidential, two types of ADA- injured worker charges can be expected to increase.

The first group is injured workers who want to work but believe they have been denied employment or return to work because of a present, past, or perceived workplace injury or predisposition to injury. These individuals would rather work than receive workers' compensation benefits. In this category would be workers who were involuntarily discharged after an injury while on leave, or who were not permitted to return to work, or who were denied a reasonable accommodation. This group also includes applicants for employment with histories of prior workplace accidents and compensation claims as well as applicants who have a job offer withdrawn because a preemployment medical examination reveals a medical condition that the employer fears will cause future injury.

A second group of charges will likely be filed by injured workers in an attempt to increase the total amount of any workers' compensation settlement. These individuals do not wish to return to work, but would rather receive the maximum amount of benefits possible. To such individuals, the ADA becomes a second avenue for relief. These workers may file a workers' compensation claim and an ADA charge knowing that in many instances the employer will settle both claims in one settlement, the amount of which is increased by the existence of the ADA charge.

Rehabilitation professionals assisting injured workers should appreciate that the ADA represents a significant change in the approach to the rehabilitation of injured workers. To understand the workers' compensation–ADA connection and its implications for rehabilitation professionals, this chapter begins by exploring the theoretical and practical interactions between workers' compensation and the ADA, including the different standards for determining who is disabled and who is entitled to compensation or damages, under the two statutes. Next, the chapter briefly discusses how the ADA changes the workplace to assist the rehabilitation psychologist to intervene in the process that turns impairments into disabilities. Finally, it explores some positive and negative implications for rehabilitation professionals of this interaction.

Theoretical Premises Underlying Both Systems

The ADA is a Federal civil rights statute which bans employment discrimination on the basis of disability against a qualified individual with a disability. Workers' compensation provides compensation for personal injury, death by accident, or illness, arising out of or in the course of employment, including medical expenses, rehabilitation, lost wages and earning capacity. The ADA does not compensate persons with disabilities for costs associated with disability; it provides redress for injury resulting from employer discrimination. This may include back pay, compensatory and punitive damages, reinstatement or hiring, restoration of benefits, reasonable accommodation and attorneys' fees.

The ADA rests on the premise that disability does not necessarily mean inability to work; it focuses upon how reasonable accommodation can remove barriers to employment caused by the interaction between functional limitations and the workplace. Workers' compensation rests on the contrasting premise that impairments are the cause of work limitations. Under workers' compensation, an employee must prove that s/he has lost wages or earning capacity because of an injury arising out of employment. In most states, however, an employer has no obligation to make any modification or reasonable accommodation to enable the worker to return to productive employment.

The ADA's key provisions and how they relate to injured workers are discussed below.

The ADA's Definition of "Disability" Differs from the Definition of an Injured Worker for Compensation Purposes

Under workers' compensation, any work caused injury or illness can be compensable; in most cases, this means only the provision of appropriate medical care and a brief period of time off from work during recovery. The ADA contains a definition of "disability" that is both more restrictive and more expansive.

"Disability" is defined in three ways by the ADA:

1. Any person who has a physical or mental impairment that substantially limits one or more of the individual's major life activities.

2. Any person who has a "record of" a substantially limiting impairment.

3. Any person who is "regarded as" having a substantially limiting impairment, regardless of whether the person is actually disabled.

A work-caused injury must substantially limit a person's major life activities in order for a worker to be "disabled" under the first part of the definition. Major life activities include caring for oneself, performing manual tasks, walking, seeing, hearing, speaking, learning, and working. (29 C. F. R. §1630. 2(i) (1992).) Other common daily activities such as sitting, standing, bending, reaching, grasping, concentrating, reasoning, and basic socialization skills would also be included.

Minor, nonchronic impairments of short duration with little or no permanent or long-term impact will not constitute a disability. This includes common workplace injuries such as a broken leg or sprained joints. (29 C. F. R. Part 1630, App. at 407 (1992).)

However, even a temporary condition, such as a broken leg, can become a disability if it takes significantly longer to heal than normal and during that time the individual is unable to walk or if the impairment heals, but leaves a permanent limp that substantially limits the individual's ability to walk. (Equal Employment Opportunity Commission, 1992, p. IX-2.)

An injured worker has a "record of" a disability when s/he has recovered in whole or in part from an impairment that had substantially limited a major life activity in the past. For example, an injured worker who had been unable to work for nine months because of a workplace accident would probably have a record of a disability. If an employer refused to hire or return this person to work because of this record, this would violate the ADA if the worker was qualified. Note, however, that a mere record of having filed a workers' compensation claim does not give a person a "record of" a substantially limiting impairment. (Equal Employment Opportunity Commission, 1992, p. IX-2.)

When an employer perceives an injured worker to be significantly restricted in the ability to perform manual tasks or any other major life activity, the injured worker is regarded as disabled by the employer. This is true whether or not the worker is, in fact, substantially limited by an impairment.

The "regarded as" part of the ADA's definition of disability is expansive and depends upon the attitude of the employer, not the nature of the injury. Many injured workers will be protected by the ADA as a result of employer's fears concerning the risk of future injury, increases in workers' compensation premiums or the cost of accommodation. These common employer concerns about injured workers create ADA coverage when it is shown that as a result, an employer took an adverse employment action because it regards an individual to be substantially limited in any major life activity such as performing manual tasks or performing a class of jobs. (Equal Employment Opportunity Commission, 1992, p. IX-3.)

"Qualified Individual with a Disability" vs. Permanent and Total Disability

Under the ADA, a "qualified individual with a disability" protected from employment discrimination is an individual with a disability who satisfies all of a job's prerequisites such as education, experience, and licenses and who can perform the job's essential functions, with or without a reasonable accommodation. Because the ADA's focus is enabling employment rather than providing benefits, the law requires employers to forgive the performance of a marginal task if a disabled worker is able to perform the fundamental tasks of a job. A job analysis can be useful in determining essential functions, but some forms of job analysis are more helpful than others in this endeavor. The EEOC's Technical Assistance Manual explains:

The job analysis may contain information on the manner in which a job currently is performed, but should not conclude that ability to perform the job in that manner is an essential function, unless there is no other way to perform the function without causing undue hardship. A job analysis will be most helpful for purposes of the ADA if it focuses on the results or outcome of a function, not solely on the way it customarily is performed. (Equal Employment Opportunity Commission, 1992, pp. II-20 to II-21.)

The ADA also recognizes that a person's disability may keep the person from performing essential job functions in the manner that they are customarily performed. The requirement to provide a reasonable accommodation responds to this problem and is discussed more fully below. Reasonable accommodation is built into the definition of a "qualified individual with a disability" in recognition that a person who is unqualified because of a disability may become qualified with accommodation.

Workers' compensation laws typically determine who is "qualified" for benefits in a very different manner. For example, in California employees are entitled to benefits if a workplace injury precludes them from engaging in their usual and customary occupation or the position in which they were engaged at the time of injury. (California Labor Code §4635(a).) Under California law, a job analysis for workers' compensation purposes documents the physical components of each job task as that job is customarily performed or was performed by a worker at the time of injury. A physician determines whether there is any job task that can no longer be performed because of the workplace injury. If so, the person is eligible for benefits and vocational rehabilitation. No consideration is given to whether the task that cannot be performed is marginal or essential to the job or whether any form of accommodation may enable the worker to perform his or her old job or a new position to which s/he can be reassigned, in spite of the injury (Wulz, 1993, p. 6). The difference in legal standards between a benefits statute and a civil rights statute can lead to a seemingly impossible result: an employee who is simultaneously permanently and totally disabled for workers' compensation purposes and yet under the ADA, be a "qualified individual with a disability."

Reasonable Accommodation and the Injured Worker

Workers' compensation law generally does not require an employer to modify a job, provide light duty or provide any equipment to enable an injured worker to return to work. Some states, including California, hold that such activities are preferred but are not required (Wulz, 1993, p. 6.).

The ADA contains a much more extensive and powerful reasonable accommodation mandate. A reasonable accommodation under the ADA means:

   i. Modifications or adjustments to a job application process that enable a qualified applicant with a disability to be considered for the position such qualified applicant desires; or

  ii. Modifications or adjustments to the work environment, or to the manner or circumstances under which the position held or desired is customarily performed, that enable a qualified individual with a disability to perform the essential functions of that position; or

 iii. Modifications or adjustments that enable a covered entity's employee with a disability to enjoy equal benefits and privileges of employment as are enjoyed by its other similarly situated employees without disabilities. (29 C.F.R. §1630.2(o)(1) (1992).)

The statute and regulations provide the following nonexclusive list of examples:

   i. Making existing facilities used by employees readily accessible to and usable by individuals with disabilities; and

  ii. Job restructuring; part-time or modified work schedules; reassignment to a vacant position; acquisition or modifications of equipment or devices; appropriate adjustment or modifications of examinations, training materials, or policies; the provision of qualified readers or interpreters; and other similar accommodations for individuals with disabilities.

Additional unpaid leave also may be a form of reasonable accommodation. In conjunction with an employer's new duty under the Family and Medical Leave Act, an employer may have to provide more than 12 weeks of unpaid leave where needed for a person with a disability.

The EEOC explained the relationship between reasonable accommodation and "light duty" in its Technical Assistance Manual, as follows:

The ADA does not require an employer to create a "light duty" position unless the "heavy duty" tasks an injured worker can no longer perform are marginal job functions which may be reallocated to co-workers as part of the reasonable accommodation of job-restructuring. In some cases, however, "light duty" positions may involve a totally different job from the job that a worker performed before the injury. Creating such positions by job restructuring is not required by the ADA. However, if an employer already has a vacant light duty position for which an injured worker is qualified, it might be a reasonable accommodation to reassign the worker to that position. If the position was created as a temporary job, a reassignment to that position need only be for a temporary period. (Equal Employment Opportunity Commission, 1992, p. IX-5.)

Providing reasonable accommodation is an interactive process between an employer and a person with a disability requesting it. The EEOC has suggested that the following steps be taken when an employee is unable to suggest a reasonable accommodation that an employer is willing to provide.

1) Identify the purpose and functions of the job the individual is seeking to perform.

2) Identify barriers to employment by consulting with the individual with a disability to ascertain his/her abilities and limitations as they relate to performance of the job's essential functions.

3) Identify possible accommodations by consulting with the individual and, where necessary, seek technical assistance.

4) Select a reasonable accommodation that is effective, and that provides an equal employment opportunity.

Undue Hardship

An employer does not have to provide a reasonable accommodation that would impose "significant difficulty or expense" on the employer in relation to its business and the resources available to provide the accommodation. (42 U.S.C. §12111(10) (1992); 29 C.F.R. §1630.2(p) (1992).) An accommodation is not required if it is "unduly costly, extensive, substantial, or disruptive, or that would fundamentally alter the nature or operation of the business." (29 C.F.R. Part 1630, App. at 413 (1992).)

Medical Screening and Health and Safety Standards

In addition to providing injured workers with an opportunity to make one more claim, doomsayers have predicted that the ADA will have catastrophic results because of its impact on medical screening. As medical costs have continued to skyrocket, many employers adopted or strengthened medical and safety standards to reduce the likelihood of workplace injuries. One aspect of this approach is to attempt to screen out applicants who pose an increased risk of injury and benefit utilization. Preemployment medical examinations have been required for several purposes including to limit job offers to persons with medical restrictions. Some employers utilized the services of third parties to research publicly available state workers' compensation files to ascertain whether an applicant had previously been injured on the job and to get information such as the body part affected and the amount of time lost. In enacting the ADA, Congress determined that the practice of making extensive disability inquiries on application forms and in interviews as well as the use of medical screening examinations had resulted in many persons with hidden disabilities being denied employment. The ADA and the EEOC's implementing regulations greatly restrict an employer's ability to make disability inquiries and require medical examinations.

Before a job offer is made, an employer may not inquire about an applicant's disability status or medical history including inquiries about past on-the-job injuries or workers' compensation claims. (42 U.S.C. §12112(d) (1992); 29 C.F.R. §1630.13 (1992).) This includes inquiries of third parties about an applicant's workers' compensation history.

An employer may condition a job offer on the satisfactory completion of a medical examination or medical inquiry provided such examination /inquiry is made of all applicants for the same job category and the results are kept confidential, with a few narrow exceptions. (42 U. S. C. §12112(d)(3) (1992); 29 C. F. R. §1630. 14 (1992).)

A job offer may be withdrawn only if the medical examination reveals that the individual is either (1) unable to do the essential functions of a job even with reasonable accommodation or (2) the individual would pose a direct threat to his/her own health or safety or the health or safety of others that cannot be eliminated or reduced by reasonable accommodation. (42 U.S.C. §12112(d)(3) (1992); 29 C.F.R. §1630.14(b) and .15 (1992).)

Medical examinations and inquiries of current employees are required to be job-related and consistent with business necessity. (42 U.S.C. §12112(d)(4) (1992); 29 C.F.R. §1630.14(c) and 1630.15 (1992).) Accordingly, return to work physical examinations must be narrowly tailored to ascertain whether the injured worker can safely perform the essential functions of his/her job with or without reasonable accommodation.

Direct Threat to Health and Safety

In order to withdraw a job offer on health or safety grounds, an employer must show that the individual poses a high probability of substantial harm to health or safety and that the risk of substantial harm cannot be eliminated or reduced below the direct threat level by a reasonable accommodation. (42 U. S. C. §12113(b) (1992); 29 C. F. R. §1630. 15(b)(2) (1992).) This is a very stringent standard that employers will not be able to meet in most circumstances. In fact, medical science will rarely have the data to demonstrate that there is a "high probability" that something bad will happen. Moreover, such claims cannot be speculative or based on future risk. Only the current abilities of the individual to safely per-form essential job functions can be assessed.

Examples:

1) An applicant for a laborer job has had no back pain or injuries in his previous jobs which require heavy lifting. But, a back X-ray reveals a back anomaly. The company doctor worries that there is a slight chance that the applicant could develop back prob-lems in the future. The threat of future back injury is too slight to meet the direct threat standard.

2) A significant risk would exist for an individual with a back anomaly who has a history of repeated back injuries in similar jobs, and whose back condition has been aggravated further by injury, and where there are no accommodations that would eliminate or reduce the risk.

3) A physician's evaluation indicates that an employee has a disc condition that might worsen in eight to ten years. This is not a sufficient indication of imminent potential harm. (Equal Employment Opportunity Commission, 1992, p. p. IV-1 to IV-17.)

Workers' compensation law provides little similar protection. Some states prohibit retaliation against a worker for filing a workers' compen-sation claim. State law also may contain a provision that penalizes an employer from returning an injured worker to a job that will likely cause new or further injury under a much lower standard of risk than that contained in the ADA's direct threat standard. The EEOC Technical Assistance Manual notes:

Some state workers' compensation statutes make an employer liable for paying additional benefits if an injury occurs because the employer assigned a person to a position likely to jeopardize the person's health or safety, or exacerbate an earlier workers' compen-sation injury. Some of these laws may permit or require an employ-er to exclude a disabled individual from employment in cases where the ADA would not permit such exclusion. In these cases, the ADA takes precedence over the state law. An employer could not assert, as a valid defense to a charge of discrimination, that it failed to hire or return to work an individual with a disability because doing so would violate a state workers' compensation law that required exclusion of this individual. (Equal Employment Opportunity Commission, 1992, p. IX-7.)

The Benefits and Pitfalls of the ADA for Workers' Compensation

The ADA will result in significant positive changes to the workers' compensation system and practices benefiting both employers and injured workers. A greater emphasis on return to work strategies and reasonable accommodation should enable injured workers to come back to work sooner. This approach reduces benefit costs, increases productivity, improves employee morale, and helps to avoid ADA charges. Community Hospitals of Central California, Inc., in Fresno, California, instituted a combined ADA compliance and workers' compensation cost containment program in 1991 with dramatic results. In 1990, its workers' compensation program costs were $2.764 million. In 1992, the program cost $1.1 million.

The company reduced its number of lost productive days from over 5,000 to under 1,500 days. And the average cost of a closed workers' compensation claim has declined from $1,525 to $468.

On the other hand, the ADA creates potentially expensive pitfalls for traditional approaches to cost containment which seek to exclude individuals who pose increased risk of benefit utilization from the workplace. ADA compliance is critical in any cost containment program because of the ADA's prohibitions against pre-offer disability inquiries and medical examinations; the stringent "direct threat" standard; the duty to accommodate including consideration of reassignment; and the availability of jury trials and compensatory and punitive damages.

Because the ADA requirements steer employers toward accommodating injured workers rather than discharging or refusing to hire them, there may be less resistance to systemic reforms that require or provide greater incentive for return to work.

The ADA's Benefits and Pitfalls for the Rehabilitation Psychologist and Other Rehabilitation Professionals

The ADA is already affecting the rehabilitation profession in a variety of ways. In the past, rehabilitation focused on changing the person with a disability to match the perceived demands of the workplace. Physical and attitudinal barriers were acknowledged, but there was little the rehabilitation professional could do to change those obstacles to placement. Today, in the post-ADA era, employers are undergoing habilitation while persons with disabilities are receiving rehabilitation.

Employer experience with accommodating existing employees who become disabled and the changing demographics indicating a shortage of qualified workers entering the labor force, both point to long-term greater receptivity for the rehabilitation professional seeking to place a qualified person with a disability. Employers will also need help from professionals knowledgeable about disability, work and accommodation. Skilled professionals have an expanded market in which to assist employers with disability-related employment issues. Some change in attitude on the part of many rehabilitation counselors will also be required. In the past, it was not unusual to get a call from a rehabilitation counselor asking whether an employer had "any jobs for handicapped people. " The ADA erases forever the concept that the rehabilitation profession should match disabilities with jobs; that there are jobs that are "good" for people who use wheelchairs or "bad" for people with hearing or vision impairments. Individualization and matching a person's abilities with job qualifications on a case-by-case basis is now the clear standard.

The rehabilitation psychologist in particular also benefits from the ADA. The workers' compensation-ADA connection creates additional emphasis on the psychology of disability. Professionals in all parts of the field of disability have long recognized that "disability" is not purely or even necessarily largely a matter of medical impairment. Whether a person's impairment becomes a "disability" depends on a wide range of family, social, economic, and psychological circumstances. Benefit programs, by their very nature, force the applicant to focus on his or her limitations. This is particularly true of the workers' compensation claims process:

> From the day the worker is injured, the claims process tries to evaluate "how disabled" the worker is. Every question they answer, every form that doctors fill out, focuses on what the worker is unable to do. The worker is put into the position of having to prove (justify) his or her situation by being incapable. While this is necessary for the evaluation of the claim, it is equally important for the worker to focus on what he or she is still capable of doing. (Pimentel, Bell, Smith, & Larson, 1993, p. 6)

The rehabilitation psychologist can play an important role in helping the injured worker to regain self-esteem and view him or herself as a person of ability, not just disability.

Rehabilitation professionals have an important role in making the promise of the ADA a reality for persons with disabilities and employers alike. Rehabilitation professionals can be the lubricant that reduces friction and improves communication between an employer and an applicant or employee with a disability. If the situation breaks down, however, a counselor can be caught in the cross-fire.

Unfortunately, just as the ADA creates opportunities for rehabilitation professionals, it also creates new liabilities and increases the likelihood that existing common-law tort liabilities will come into new prominence. Here are some of the critical unanswered questions:

1) What can a counselor tell an employer about a client's disability without violating the ADA?

2) If an employer discriminatorily refused to hire a client after he or she learned of the client's disability from the counselor, could the counselor also be liable for back pay and damages under the ADA? The Rehabilitation Services Administration issued a Technical Assistance Circular RSA-TAC-FY-93-01 instructing counselors not to advise employers of a client's disability pursuant to §504 of the Rehabilitation Act of 1973 and the ADA.

3) If the employer followed the counselor's recommendation and hired the client, and the client later hurt himself or herself, could the counselor be liable to the client for negligent failure to advise the client against taking the job? Could the counselor be liable to the employer for its workers' compensation expenses for the same reason? What if the client injures a third party because of a disability-related limitation? Could the counselor be liable to the third party?

4) What if the counselor recommends against hiring or returning a client to work because of an incorrectly perceived "direct threat" to the client or others? Is the counselor liable as an agent of the employer under the ADA? Is the counselor additionally liable under negligence law?

5) Because the ADA overrides state immunity, could a state vocational rehabilitation counselor be held individually liable for damages for violating the ADA? How much protection, if any, does state law provide a counselor?

6) Does the counselor have a duty to tell a client that an employer has discriminated against the client? Is the counselor liable to the client if the counselor fails to do so? Is he or she liable to the employer for defamation if the counselor does so?

7) Is a rehabilitation program, private or public, an "employment agency" under the ADA, responsible for compliance with the ADA in all of its activities?

Conclusion

The ADA will have a dramatic impact on how injured workers are treated under the workers' compensation system. The practical focus of employers must change from paying workers off to keep them from the workplace, to aggressively trying to return them to work. It is simply better for all concerned to pay a person to do productive work rather than pay him/her to sit at home and watch television.

This change in emphasis will not occur unless those involved in the workers' compensation system understand its ADA implications. Injured workers can be an "individual with a disability" under the ADA and qualified, with or without reasonable accommodation, to perform a job's essential functions even if they are permanently disabled for workers' compensation purposes. The ADA also will have a dramatic impact on how rehabilitation professionals work with injured workers and employers. The ADA is transforming the workplace to bring down attitudinal and structural barriers to employment of persons with disabilities. Benefit programs such as workers' compensation create their own barrier to employment by focusing the claimant and the employer on the limitations flowing from an impairment rather than the individual's remaining abilities. The rehabilitation psychologist can play an important role in enhancing an injured workers' self-esteem and self-concept as a person with abilities as well as limitations.

At the same time, the rehabilitation professional can be caught in the middle of an ADA employment dispute. For this reason, it remains critical for rehabilitation professionals to understand the ADA and the responsibilities and obligations it may impose on their profession.

References

The Equal Employment Opportunity Commission (1992). *Technical assistance manual on the employment provisions (Title I) of the Americans with Disabilities Act.* Washington, DC: Author.

Pimentel, R., Bell, C., Smith, G.M., & Larson, H. (1993). *The workers' compensation—ADA connection: Supervisory tools for workers' compensation cost containment that reduce ADA liability.* Chatsworth, CA: Milt Wright & Associates, Inc.

Wulz, S.S. (1993). A contractual relationship to discriminate. *California Workers' Compensation Enquirer, 10.*

·8·

The Alcohol and Drug Provisions
of the ADA

Implications for Employers and Employees

Nancy Jones[1]

Introduction

The Americans with Disabilities Act[2], (ADA) is a far-reaching civil rights statute protecting the civil rights of an estimated 43,000,000 Americans with disabilities.[3] The act prohibits discrimination based on disability and contains a functional definition of "individual with a disability" that could include individuals who abuse alcohol and individuals who have formerly illegally used drugs[4] if they are determined to be otherwise qualified. The inclusion of these individuals raises some complex issues regarding the rights and responsibilities of both employers and employees. This chapter will examine the history of protection against discrimination based on alcohol or drug use, the provisions of the ADA, and the changes made from prior law; and will examine these provisions with a particular emphasis on issues that are of concern to clinicians who provide alcohol and drug abuse treatment or psychologists who may be consulted by employers regarding alcohol and drug issues in the workplace. It concludes that, although the ADA has expanded protections for individuals who are alcoholics and for individuals who have formerly illegally used drugs, civil rights protections have been reduced for individuals who are currently illegally using drugs.

History of Nondiscrimination Protection Based on Alcohol or Drug Use

The ADA and its provisions relating to alcohol and drug use have their roots in the Rehabilitation Act of 1973.[5] Section 504 of the Rehabilitation Act prohibits discrimination against an otherwise qualified individual with a handicap, solely by reason of handicap, in any program or activity that receives federal financial assistance, in executive agencies, and in the U.S. Postal Service.[6] It differs from the ADA in several respects, the most significant being the scope of coverage. While section 504 is limited to the entities listed above, the ADA extends essentially the same protections of section 504 into the private sector. Starting on July 26, 1992, the ADA covered all employers with 25 or more employees. On July 26, 1994, this coverage will be expanded to reach employers with 15 to 24 employees.[7]

Section 7 of the Rehabilitation Act [8] defines the term "individual with handicaps" as used in section 504. This definition originally stated that the term meant any person who "(i) has a physical or mental impairment which substantially limits one or more of such person's major life activities, (ii) has a record of such an impairment, or (iii) is regarded as having such an impairment." Amendments made in 1978 added an additional sentence stating that for the purposes of employment, the definition "does not include any individual who is an alcoholic or drug abuser whose current use of alcohol or drugs prevents such individual from performing the duties of the job in question or whose employment, by reason of such current alcohol or drug abuse, would constitute a direct threat to property or the safety of others."

The definition of "individual with handicaps" under the Rehabilitation Act is a functional one and does not attempt to list the various conditions that might be covered. This has led to some confusion over what conditions are, in fact, covered under section 504. When the Secretary of Health, Education and Welfare (HEW) was formulating regulations for section 504 in 1976, prior to the 1978 amendments, the issue of the coverage of individuals who abused alcohol or drugs was raised in a request for public comments.[9] An opinion was sought from the Attorney General who concluded that such individuals were covered under section 504 if they were discriminated against solely because of their status as individuals who abused drugs or alcohol.[10] In arriving at this conclusion, the Attorney General examined the legislative history of the Rehabilitation Act and found that although Congress had not specifically discussed the issue, the implications of the legislative history supported coverage.

However, in order to be covered with regard to employment under section 504, an individual must be "otherwise qualified." The Attorney General specifically stated that:

> "our conclusion that alcoholic and drug addicts are 'handicapped individuals' for purposes of section 504 does not mean that such a person must be hired or permitted to participate in a federally assisted program if the manifestations of his conditions prevent him from effectively performing the job in question or participation would be unduly disruptive to others, and section 504 presumably

would not require unrealistic accommodation in such a situation."[11]

Similarly, the Attorney General did not read section 504 as prohibiting the application of reasonable rules of conduct to such individuals, such as a prohibition of possession or use of alcohol or drugs while on the premises of an employer. In conclusion, the Attorney General noted:

"the statute does not require the impossible. It does not unrealistically require that recipients of Federal contracts and grants ignore all the behavioral or other problems that may accompany a person's alcoholism or drug addiction if they interfere with the performance of his job or his effective participation in a federally assisted program. At the same time, the statute requires that contractors and grantees covered by the Act not automatically deny employment or benefits to persons solely because they might find their status as alcoholics or drug addicts personally offensive, any more than contractors or grantees could discriminate against an individual who had some other condition or disease—such as cancer, multiple sclerosis, amputation, or blindness—unless its manifestations or his conduct rendered him ineligible."[12]

As a result of the Attorney General's opinion, the final section 504 regulations of the Department of Health, Education, and Welfare included individuals who abused alcohol or drugs within the definition of "individual with handicaps." In the appendix to the regulations, the findings of the Attorney General were emphasized and it was observed that:

"[a] recipient may hold a drug addict or alcoholic to the same standard of performance and behavior to which it holds others, even if any unsatisfactory performance or behavior is related to the person's drug addiction or alcoholism. In other words, while an alcoholic or drug addict may not be denied services or disqualified from employment solely because of his or her condition, the behavioral manifestations of the condition may be taken into account in determining whether he or she is qualified."[13]

Despite the careful explanations of the conditions under which individuals who abuse alcohol or drugs were covered under section 504, the inclusion of these individuals in the HEW regulations raised considerable concern, especially among employers. Congress acted to assuage this concern in passing the Rehabilitation Act Amendments of 1978.[14] These amendments added an additional sentence to the definition of handicapped person: "[f]or purposes of sections 503 and 504 as such sections relate to employment, such term does not include any individual who is an alcoholic or drug abuser whose current use of alcohol or drugs prevents such individual from performing the duties of the job in question or whose employment, by reason of such current alcohol or drug abuse, would constitute a direct threat to property or the safety of others." This addition has been seen as "formaliz[ing] the Attorney General's view that behavioral effects of current alcohol or drug use may disqualify alcoholics or drug addicts from the protections of the Act in regard to employment." (Burgdorf, 1980)

The legislative history of the 1978 amendments also supports this view. Senator Williams stated that the "amendment is designed to clear up some misunderstandings about the employment rights of alcoholics and drug addicts under the Act, and to make absolutely clear that employers covered by the Act must not discriminate against those persons having a history or condition of alcoholism or drug abuse who are qualified for the particular employment they seek."[15] The House Conference Report specifically observed that "[t]he conference substitute clarifies that only those active alcoholics or drug abusers who cannot perform the essential functions of a job in question or who present a danger to life and property are not covered by the employment provisions of section 503 and 504."[16] The explanation of the conference report given in the Senate further elaborated on the intent of Congress concerning this section. It noted that the "legislative history of the 1973 Act, as authoritatively interpreted by the Attorney General, made clear that qualified individuals with conditions or histories of alcoholism or drug addiction were protected from discrimination by covered employments...."[17] This intention was praised as in keeping with the experience of professionals that 'many recovered alcoholics or drug abusers perform competently and reliably...' and it was noted that "[m]any large corporations have recognized that simply firing or refusing to hire an individual fighting an alcohol problem is not only bad social policy, but in the long run also exacerbates their economic losses due to alcoholism."[18] Senator Williams also emphasized that employers do not have to indiscriminately hire persons with histories or conditions of alcoholism or addiction, "but are obliged to hire and retain only those who are qualified with respect to performance, behavior, and other job-related criteria."[19] In addition, Senator Williams noted that an individual whose current alcohol or drug use poses a direct threat to the safety of human beings or to property is not protected by the Act.

The rationale for including individuals who abuse alcohol or drugs in the coverage of section 504 was examined in the Senate debates where it was emphasized that there is substantial authority for the proposition that alcoholism and drug addiction are physical and/or mental impairments. Senator Hathaway observed that "the Rehabilitation Act expresses a general preference, in terms of social costs and the quality of individual lives, for reintegrating the handicapped into productive society, rather than shunting them aside and spending millions for poor custodial care. There is no reason to reverse that preference where alcoholics or drug abusers are concerned."[20] Senator Williams noted that employment is often critical in providing the stability necessary for rehabilitation and that "[m]any 'active' alcoholics and drug addicts hold jobs and perform them satisfactorily."[21] Judicial decisions after the 1978 amendments generally followed this rationale.[22]

In summary, section 504, as interpreted by the Attorney General, clarified by the 1978 amendments, and interpreted by the courts, considered alcoholism and drug addictions as physical or mental impairments. As such, individuals with those impairments could be discriminated against in employment only if the impairments actually rendered them unqualified for the position or posed a danger. The emphasis was not on the label but rather on the actual abilities of the individual.

Employers still harbored fears concerning the employment of individuals who abuse alcohol or drugs, and amendments were proposed at various times to change the coverage of section 504. These were not successful until the passage of the ADA, an Act which rightfully is hailed as expanding the rights of individuals with disabilities but which actually limits some of those rights with regard to individuals who use illegal drugs.

Statutory Provisions of the Americans with Disabilities Act

The ADA contains the same expansive functional definition of "individual with a disability" that is used for section 504. "The term 'disability' means, with respect to an individual—(A) a physical or mental impairment that substantially limits one or more of the major life activities of such individual; (B) a record of such an impairment; or (C) being regarded as having such an impairment."[23] However, the politics of passage added certain exceptions to this definition. Transvestites were specifically excluded from coverage twice in the statutory language of the ADA.[24] Other conditions such as pedophilia, exhibitionism, voyeurism, and other sexual behavior disorders also were excluded.[25] Although many of these disorders may not have met the criteria of "substantially limiting one or more...major life impairments" there was considerable concern in the Congress about negative public reaction to a prohibition of discrimination against people with conditions that often raise moral concerns.

Like sexual disorders, drug abuse issues were a political "hot potato." A specific section in the ADA was added to deal with the illegal use of drugs. It states:

a) In General—For purposes of this Act, the term "individual with a disability" does not include an individual who is currently engaging in the illegal use of drugs, when the covered entity acts on the basis of such use.

b) Rules of Construction—Nothing in subsection (a) shall be construed to exclude as an individual with a disability an individual who

(1) has successfully completed a supervised drug rehabilitation program and is no longer engaging in the illegal use of drugs, or has otherwise been rehabilitated successfully and is no longer engaging in such use;

(2) is participating in a supervised rehabilitation program and is no longer engaging in such use; or

(3) is erroneously regarded as engaging in such use, but is not engaging in such use;

except that it shall not be a violation of this Act for a covered entity to adopt or administer reasonable policies or procedures, including but not limited to drug testing, designed to ensure that an individual described in paragraph (1) or (2) is no longer engaging in the illegal use of drugs; however, nothing in this section shall be construed to encourage, prohibit, restrict, or authorize the conducting of testing for the illegal use of drugs.

c) Health and Other Services—Notwithstanding subsection (a) and section 511(b)(3), an individual shall not be denied health services or services provided in connection with drug rehabilitation, on the basis of the current illegal use of drugs if the individual is otherwise entitled to such services.

d) Definition of Illegal Use of Drugs—

(1) In general—The term "illegal use of drugs" means the use of drugs, the possession or distribution of which is unlawful under the Controlled Substances Act (21 U.S.C. 811). Such term does not include the use of a drug taken under supervision by a licensed health care professional, or other uses authorized by the Controlled Substances Act or other provisions of Federal law.

(2) Drugs—The term "drug" means a controlled substance as defined in schedules I through V of section 202 of the Controlled Substance Act.[26]

A similar section specifically relating to employment is contained in Title I of the ADA. It states that for the purposes of Title I, the term "qualified individual with a disability" shall not include an employee or applicant who is currently engaging in the illegal use of drugs, when the covered entity acts on the basis of such use."[27] The rules of construction for the Title I provision are the same as those quoted above. In addition, though, the Title I provision specifically lists several actions a covered entity may take. A covered employer "(1) may prohibit the illegal use of drugs and the use of alcohol at the workplace by all employees; (2) may require that employees shall not be under the influence of alcohol or be engaging in the illegal use of drugs at the workplace; (3) may require that employees behave in conformance with the requirements established under the Drug-Free Workplace Act of 1988 (41 U.S.C. sec. 701 et seq.); (4) may hold an employee who engages in the illegal use of drugs or who is an alcoholic to the same qualification standards for employment or job performance and behavior that such entity holds other employees, even if any unsatisfactory performance or behavior is related to the drug use or alcoholism of such employee; and (5) may, with respect to Federal regulations regarding alcohol and the illegal use of drugs..." make certain requirements for compliance with Department of Defense, Nuclear Regulatory Commission, and Department of Transportation regulations.[28] The Title I provisions also provide that a test to determine the illegal use of drugs is not to be considered a medical examination for the purposes of Title I. Therefore, it is not a violation of the ADA to conduct drug testing for applicants and employees.[29]

The ADA added a section amending the Rehabilitation Act to conform its requirements to that of the ADA. This section contained essentially the same language as the ADA but also added a subsection relating to educational services and contained a specific subsection excluding individuals who are alcoholic "whose current use of alcohol prevents such individual from performing the duties of the job in question or whose employment, by reason of such current alcohol abuse, would constitute a direct threat to property or the safety of others."[30]

The ADA contains very similar but arguably somewhat different requirements. Under the ADA, an individual with a disability must be able to perform the essential functions of the job which has been defined as meaning "the fundamental job duties of the employment position the individual with a disability holds or desires."[31] In addition, the direct threat language differs from that in the ADA. The ADA's statutory language refers to a "direct threat to the health or safety of others in the workplace."[32] Although the EEOC's regulations expanded upon this to include a "direct threat to the health or safety of the individual or others in the workplace,"[33] neither the ADA's statutory language or the EEOC's regulations contain a reference to a direct threat to property.

Statutory Analysis

Thus, currently under both the ADA and section 504 of the Rehabilitation Act, an individual who illegally uses drugs is not covered. An employer can discriminate against such an individual on the basis of current drug use without violating either statute. There is no protection provided for relapses during the course of rehabilitation; the salient factor concerning ADA protection is the use of drugs. Under the ADA, an individual is either a former illegal drug user, and therefore covered, or a current illegal drug user, and therefore not entitled to any protections. An individual who has a relapse while undergoing treatment for a drug problem, is not protected by the ADA at the time of the relapse, even if the relapse is of short duration and does not affect job performance. The implications of this approach could be quite significant for persons in treatment. Although it is easy to be placed into the category of a "current user" due to a relapse, it is much more difficult to be placed into the protected category of a "former user." There is no time frame specified, and the discussion in the legislative history indicates that coverage is denied if the illegal use of a drug occurred recently enough to justify a reasonable belief that a person's drug use is current.[34] Therefore, an individual could be excluded from the ADA's coverage due to a relapse and fired from his or her job, without triggering a violation of the act. This rather extreme consequence could easily lead the individual who suffers a relapse to discontinue treatment or to be less than honest with the counselor.

This approach differs significantly from the former coverage in section 504, under which drug use was not an automatic disqualification if the individual was found to be otherwise qualified for the job. Previously, under section 504, individuals who currently used drugs were seen as having a medical problem that warranted an adverse action only where the individual presented a danger or was unable to perform the duties of the job in question. Present law takes a more punitive approach to the current illegal use of drugs.

However, if an individual is a recovered illegal drug user or an active or recovered alcoholic, the individual is covered by the ADA or section 504 to the same extent as other disabled individuals. These categories may enable the individual to meet the first criteria for finding discrimination—that of fitting the definition of an individual with a disability — but the individual must also meet other criteria. To have a successful case under the ADA and section 504, the individuals must be otherwise qualified for the employment—with or without reasonable accommodation that does not constitute an undue hardship to the employer—and must not pose a direct threat to themselves or others. For example, an individual with severe visual impairments would not be qualified for a position as a bus driver and an employer would not be required to hire such an individual for that position. That example is an easy one; the terms "otherwise qualified," "reasonable accommodation," "undue hardship," and "direct threat," are complicated, and their application to particular situations involving drug or alcohol abuse are not always clear. Although each of these terms has been the subject of extensive articles, (Cooper, 1991; Crespi, 1990; Gardner & Campanella, 1991; Holtzman, Jennings, & Schenck, 1992; Postol & Kadue, 1991; Shaller, 1991; Shaller & Rosen, 1991, 1992; Weirich, 1991) it would be helpful to examine these concepts briefly and analyze how they might apply to the situations posed by individuals who abuse drugs or alcohol.

Qualified Individual with a Disability

As was noted above, the employment title of the ADA contains a specific definition of "qualified individual with a disability." This definition does little more than reiterate the fact that an individual who currently is using drugs illegally is not covered under the act. The regulations promulgated by the Equal Employment Opportunity Commission (EEOC) are more specific. A qualified individual with a disability "means an individual with a disability who satisfies the requisite skill, experience, education and other job-related requirements of the employment position such individual holds or desires, and who, with or without reasonable accommodation, can perform the essential functions of the position."[35] Essential functions are further defined in the EEOC regulations as "the fundamental job duties of the employment position the individual holds or desires" and do not include the marginal functions of the position.[36] For example, an individual with an alcohol or substance abuse problem who applies for a position as a lawyer must have a legal education and be able to perform legal duties, such as appearances in court, filing of timely briefs, and completion of competent research. An individual who does not meet the specific essential requirements of the job would not be otherwise qualified. The question then becomes whether a reasonable accommodation that does not impose an undue hardship would enable such an individual to perform the job.

Reasonable Accommodation

Reasonable accommodation is defined in Title I of the ADA as including, "(A) making existing facilities used by employees readily accessible to and usable by individuals with disabilities; and (B) job restructuring, part-time or modified work schedules, reassignment to a vacant position, acquisition or modification of equipment or devices, appropriate adjustment or modifications of examinations, training materials or policies, the provision of qualified readers or interpreters, and other similar accommodations for individuals with disabilities."[37] Many of these statutory examples are more appropriate for disabilities other than alcohol or drug abuse;

however, several of them could be useful for individuals with an alcohol or substance abuse problem. Many of these individuals find it necessary to receive regular counseling or attend meetings such as Alcoholics Anonymous. An employer may well be required to restructure a job position so as to allow attendance at the meetings or time for individual therapy. In addition, it might also be required that an employer allow groups such as Alcoholics Anonymous to meet in the employer's workspace if workspace is provided to other employee groups such as a book club.[38] A clinician who is providing treatment to an individual with an alcohol or substance abuse problem may be asked by the individual to provide supporting documentation to the employer for such accommodations. A clinician who receives requests directly from the employer would need to be sensitive to confidentiality issues and the privacy concerns of the individual involved. However, regardless of the clinician's statements regarding the necessity of various accommodations, whether these accommodations would be required would depend upon whether they would create an undue hardship on the employer.

Undue Hardship

It is considered to be discrimination under Title I of the ADA, if an employer refuses to make a reasonable accommodation to the known physical or mental limitations of an otherwise qualified individual with a disability who is an applicant or employee, unless the covered entity can demonstrate that the accommodation would impose an undue hardship on the operation of the employer's business.[39] Undue hardship is defined in the statute as meaning "an action requiring significant difficulty or expense, when considered in light of (specified) factors...." The factors to be considered include: "(i) the nature and cost of the accommodation needed under this Act; (ii) the overall financial resources of the facility or facilities involved in the provision of the reasonable accommodation; the number of persons employed at such facility; the effect on expenses and resources, or the impact otherwise of such accommodation upon the operation of the facility; (iii) the overall financial resources of the covered entity; the overall size of the business of a covered entity with respect to the number of its employees; the number, type, and location of its facilities; and (iv) the type of operation or operations of the covered entity, including the composition, structure, and functions of the workforce of such entity; the geographic separateness, administrative, or fiscal relationship of the facility or facilities in question to the covered entity."[40]

The legislative history of the undue hardship provision indicates that the factors to be considered were not intended to be an exhaustive list;

rather "it is intended to provide general guidance about the nature of the obligation."[41] Like other provisions of the ADA, the interpretation of what is an appropriate reasonable accommodation and what does or does not constitute an undue hardship is determined by an examination of the specific facts in a particular situation. For example, a large corporation with a large physical plant may be required to allow employees to use a room for Alcoholics Anonymous meetings, while a small retail business employing 15 persons may not be so required. Similarly, in certain positions, such as many office jobs, regular time off to attend therapy sessions may be required as a reasonable accommodation. However, such an accommodation may pose an undue hardship in certain situations; for example, when a nurse employed by a small health care facility is legally required to be on-site at all times, or when a worker in an assembly line can only be replaced at specific times.

Direct Threat

In order to be considered to be a qualified individual with a disability, an individual must not pose a "direct threat." The term is statutorily defined as meaning "a significant risk to the health or safety of others that cannot be eliminated by reasonable accommodation."[42] This is a limitation on coverage that is of key importance to individuals who are alcoholics or who are substance abusers. There certainly are scenarios where the employment of an individual who has an alcohol problem is inappropriate. For example, positions involving driving a train or flying an airplane would necessitate abstinence from alcohol use while such duties are being performed. The statutory provisions of the ADA as quoted above clearly allow for the prohibition of alcohol use in certain positions such as those covered by relevant regulations of the Department of Defense, the Nuclear Regulatory Commission, and the Department of Transportation.[43] An individual can be considered to pose a direct threat even where not specifically covered by these regulations.

The ADA regulations promulgated by the EEOC provide more specific guidance about how a determination of a direct threat is to be made. The regulations specifically add to the statutory language by defining direct threat as meaning a significant risk of substantial harm to the health or safety of the individual or others that cannot be eliminated by reasonable accommodation.[44] The addition of the phrase "of the individual" was a controversial one which was criticized as paternalistic. The EEOC argued, however, that "an employer would not be required to hire an individual, disabled by narcolepsy, who frequently and unexpectedly loses consciousness for a carpentry job the essential functions of which require the use of power saws and other dangerous equipment, where no accommodation exists that will reduce or eliminate the risk."[45] A similar argument could be made with regard to an individual who drinks alcohol while on the job.

In addition to covering a direct threat to an individual, the EEOC regulations emphasize that a determination of direct threat shall be based on "an individualized assessment of the individual's present ability to safely perform the essential functions of the job."[46] This individualized assessment is to be based on "reasonable medical judgment that relies on the most current medical knowledge and/or on the best available objective evidence." Certain factors which are to be considered are "(1) The duration of the risk; (2) The nature and severity of the potential harm; (3) The likelihood that the potential harm will occur; and (4) The imminence of the potential harm."[47] As the legislative history also notes, an employer must identify the specific risk that the individual with a disability would pose, make such a determination on a case-by-case basis, and not make it based on "generalizations, misperceptions, ignorance, irrational fears, patronizing attitudes, or pernicious mythologies."[48] This requirement is of particular importance for individuals who are alcoholics or who have formerly used drugs since they may be perceived to be a threat based on ignorance or irrational fears.

A recent case under title III of the ADA relating to public accommodations illustrates how the concept of direct threat may be applied. In *Anderson v. Little League Baseball, Inc.*,[49] a little league coach who uses a wheelchair was prohibited by the organization from using the coacher's box. The organization argued that his presence on the field created a danger for the children playing the sport since they should not have the added concern of avoiding a collision with a wheelchair during their participation in the game. However, the court, noting that the coach had been performing these duties for three years with no difficulties, rejected the argument, observing that allegations of a direct threat or a danger must be based on objective evidence and not mere allegations of a risk. "An individualized inquiry is essential if the law is to achieve its goal of protecting disabled individuals from discrimination based on prejudice, stereotypes, or unfounded fear."[50] The court further noted there was no indication in the records of the case that there had been any individualized assessment or any inquiry concerning the nature, duration, and severity of the risk posed by the plaintiff; the probability that the potential injury would actually occur; or whether reasonable modifications of policies, practices or procedures would mitigate the risk.

Thus, determining whether a particular individual poses a direct threat is an area where the expertise and input of clinicians who provide alcohol and substance abuse treatment is of key importance.[51] Individualized assessments are to be made on the basis of "reasonable medical judgment." However, clinicians should offer such advice with care. Questions regarding a direct threat or dangerousness can not generally be answered with certainty and issues regarding the liability of clinicians for mistaken determinations could be raised. In *Tarasoff v. Regents of University of California*,[52] the California Supreme Court held that when a therapist determines or should determine by using professional standards that a patient presents a serious danger of violence to another, he or she has an obligation to use reasonable care to protect the intended victim. Although there is no uniformity in the judicial decisions in some subsequent cases, the *Tarasoff* decision has been extended to situations where no specific victim has been threatened[53]or where property damage, not personal injury, was at issue.[54] In *Peck v. Counseling Service of Addison County*,[55] a patient of a nonprofit counseling service told the therapist that he was angry at his father and wanted to "get back" at him by burning his barn down. The therapist extracted a promise that the patient would not burn down the barn but six days later, the barn was burned. The parents sued the counseling service and the state supreme court held that a mental health professional who knew of a serious risk of danger to an identifiable victim has a duty to exercise reasonable care to protect him or her from that danger. Although only property damage was involved here, the court emphasized that arson was a violent act and could be a threat to people.

A Tarasoff-type argument could be made against a substance abuse counselor who knew of a client's relapse, and knew that this relapse created a possible danger but stated that the individual did not pose a direct threat. For example, if a surgeon, in treatment for drug abuse suffered a relapse and told the counselor that he was still going to operate on patient John Doe, who subsequently dies as a result of the surgeon's actions, the patient's family could arguably sue the counselor under the Tarasoff theory. Counselors would be particularly at risk if they knew the client had suffered a relapse and did not mention it. This is because the use of illegal drugs is a per se disqualification from coverage under the ADA. However, this possibility of liability does not mean that a psychologist or other counselor should refrain from any interpretations regarding direct threat. Rather, blanket or absolute statements, such as "no possibility of relapse" should be avoided. A statement based on observed facts, for example, the length of term of sobriety and dedication to treatment procedures, would be considered to be a "reasonable medical judgment" and would be unlikely to result in liability for the counselor.

Current Users of Drugs

Another key issue that is likely to arise with regard to individuals who have illegally used drugs is when such individuals are no longer considered to be current drug users and therefore covered by the ADA. In other words, when are individuals considered to be "currently engaging" in the use of drugs? The ADA conference report states that the provision excluding such individuals "is not intended to be limited to persons who use drugs on the day of, or within a matter of days or weeks before, the action in question. Rather, the provision is intended to apply to a person whose illegal use of drugs occurred recently enough to justify a reasonable belief that a person's drug use is current."[56] The exact length of time that an individual is required to be drug free in order to be considered an "individual with a disability" under the ADA is not stated.

A related question is whether former drug use is ever relevant in making an employment decision. Although current users are not covered, the ADA covers individuals who are former drug users in order "to carry out our national commitment to encourage all those who need it to come forward for treatment, and to ensure that individuals who have successfully overcome drug problems will not face senseless or irrational barriers that work to impede their full reintegration into society."[57] However, this requirement has raised significant concerns, particularly in the employment offices of police departments, that convicted drug sellers or individuals who have used drugs will have to be hired. First, it should be noted that having a prison record does not constitute a disability,[58] so a police department could reject an applicant for employment on the grounds of a prison record, regardless of whether that applicant was an individual with disabilities. If an individual does not have a prison record but has used illegal drugs, it is still possible that a police department would not have to hire such an individual. "An employer, such as a law enforcement agency, may also be able to impose a qualification standard that excludes individuals with a history of illegal use of drugs if it can show that the standard is job-related and consistent with business necessity."[59] Although this guidance is helpful, it does not answer all the questions presented by this situation. The type of drug use and the exact position may be key in making the determination of whether the ADA has been violated. For example, an employer may not be able to impose an employment standard that would exclude an individual who had used illegal drugs twenty years previously and who is applying for a position as a clerk in a police department. On the other hand, an employment standard for the position of an undercover narcotics officer that excludes individuals who have used illegal drugs in the past year, would appear to be job-related.

Conclusion

The Americans with Disabilities Act provides broad-based nondiscrimination protection in the private sector for individuals with disabilities. The covered class is defined in the statute as including persons who are alcoholics or who have formerly illegally used drugs. Although discrimination against these individuals was prohibited by section 504 of the Rehabilitation Act of 1973, this section is limited to entities that receive federal financial assistance, the federal executive agencies, and the U.S. Postal Service. The expansion of nondiscrimination protection for these individuals should assist clinicians working with them by limiting the worry that employment may be lost simply due to an individual's status as an alcoholic or former illegal drug user. However, in one respect, the ADA takes a step backward from the law as it was under section 504.

The ADA's nondiscrimination protection is patterned on the medical model used by section 504 of the Rehabilitation Act of 1973, and seeks to treat such individuals as having a physical or mental impairment that should not prohibit them from employment unless they were unqualified for the position or posed a direct threat. However, the ADA's total exclusion of current drug users illustrates the ambivalence of society toward individuals who illegally use drugs. By excluding such individuals as a class, the ADA and its conforming amendments to section 504 take a regressive approach to civil rights law. Previously, section 504 had covered such individuals but only if they were otherwise qualified and posed no danger. The exclusion from employment of individuals who are qualified and do not pose a danger may greatly limit the ADA's goal of equal protection for all citizens with disabilities. An individual who is currently abusing drugs may be deterred from seeking treatment if he or she is presently employed, because he or she may be considered to be an active drug user for some unspecified time after treatment is begun. Similarly, an individual who suffers a relapse may be dismissed from employment, and may discontinue treatment as a result, due to loss of health insurance. Such disincentives for treatment harm the individual, the employer, and society in general. If the goal of integrating such individuals into society is to be accomplished, a return to the previous standard for current drug users is necessary.

Notes

[1] Legislative Attorney, American Law Division, Congressional Research Service, Library of Congress. The views expressed in this article are the views of the author, not necessarily those of the Library of Congress.

[2] P.L. 101-336, 42 U.S.C. secs. 12101 et seq.

[3] 42 U.S.C. sec. 12101.

[4] 42 U.S.C. sec. 12102; 42 U.S.C. sec. 12210.

[5] 29 U.S.C. secs. 701 et seq.

[6] 29 U.S.C. sec. 794.

[7] 42 U.S.C. sec. 12111.

[8] 29 U.S.C. sec. 706(8)(B).

[9] 41 Fed. Reg. 20296 (May 17, 1976).

[10] 43 O.A.G. No. 12 (April 12, 1977).

[11] Id.

[12] Id.

[13] 45 C.F.R. Part 84, Appendix A.

[14] Comprehensive Rehabilitation Act Amendments of 1978, P.L. 95-602.

[15] 124 Cong. Rec. 37509 (Statement of Sen. Williams).

[16] H.Conf. Rep. No. 1780, 95th Cong., 2d Sess. 102 (1978).

[17] 124 Cong. Rec. S. 19001 (Oct. 14, 1978)(Remarks of Sen. Williams).

[18] 124 Cong. Rec. S. 19001 (Oct. 14, 1978)(Remarks of Sen. Williams).

[19] Id. at 19002.

[20] 124 Cong. Rec. 30324 (1978)(Remarks of Senator Hathaway).

[21] Id. (Remarks of Sen. Williams).

[22] See e.g., Davis v. Bucher, 451 F.Supp. 791 (E.D. Pa. 1978).

[23] 42 U.S.C. sec. 12102.

[24] 42 U.S.C. sec. 12208; 42 U.S.C. sec. 12211.

[25] 42 U.S.C. sec. 12211.

[26] 42 U.S.C. sec. 12210.

[27] 42 U.S.C. sec. 12114.

[28] Id.

[29] 29 C.F.R. §1630.16(c)(1).

[30] 29 U.S.C. sec. 706(8)(C)(v).

[31] 29 C.F.R. §1630.2(n).

[32] 42 U.S.C. §12113(b).

[33] 29 C.F.R. §1630.15(b)(2).

[34] H.Conf.Rep. No. 596, 101st Cong., 2d Sess. at 64.

[35] 29 C.F.R. sec. 1630.2(m).

36 29 C.F.R. sec. 1630.2(n).

37 42 U.S.C. sec. 12111(9).

38 29 C.F.R. sec. 1630.2 (o)(1)(iii).

39 42 U.S.C. sec. 12112(10)(A).

40 42 U.S.C. sec. 12111(10)(B).

41 S. Rep. No. 116, 101st Cong, 1st Sess. 35 (1989).

42 42 U.S.C. sec. 12111.

43 42 U.S.C. sec. 12114.

44 29 C.F.R. sec. 1630.2(r).

45 56 Fed. Reg. 35745 (July 26, 1991).

46 29 C.F.R. sec. 1630.2(r).

47 Id.

48 S. Rep. No. 116, 101st Cong., 1st Sess. 27 (1989).

49 61 U.S.L.W. 2050 (D. Ariz. 1992).

50 Id.

51 56 Fed. Reg. 35745 (July 26, 1991).

52 17 Cal.3d 425, 551 P.2d 334, 131 Cal. Rptr. 14 (1976).

53 Lipari v. Sears, Roebuck & Co.,497 F. Supp. 185 (D.Neb. 1980).

54 Peck v. Counseling Service of Addison County, 146 Vt. 61, 499 A.2d 422 (1985).

55 Id.

56 H.Conf.Rep. No. 596, 101st Cong., 2d Sess. at 64.

57 135 Cong. Rec. S 10775 (daily ed. Sept. 7, 1989)(Remarks of Sen.Kennedy).

58 S.Rep. No. 116, 101st Cong. 1st Sess. 21 (1989).

59 56 Fed. Reg. 35746 (July 26, 1991).

References

Burgdorf, R. (1980). *The Legal Rights of Handicapped Persons*. Baltimore, MD: Brooks.

Cooper, J. (1991). Overcoming barriers to employment: The meaning of reasonable accommodation and undue hardship in the Americans with Disabilities Act. *139. U. Pa. L. Rev.* 1423.

Crespi, G. (1990). Efficiency rejected: Evaluating 'undue hardship' claims under the Americans with Disabilities Act. *26. Tulsa L. J.* 1.

Feldblum, C. (1991). The Americans with Disabilities Act definition of disability. *7. The Labor Lawyer* 11.

Gardner, R., & Campanella, C. (1991). The undue hardship defense to the Reasonable Accommodation Requirement of the Americans with Disabilities Act. *7. The Labor Lawyer* 37.

Holtzman, G., Jennings, K., & Schenck, D. (1992). Reasonable accommodation of the disabled worker—A job for the man or a man for the job?, *44. Baylor L. Rev.* 279.

Kemp, E., & Bell, C. (1991). A Labor Lawyer's Guide to the Americans with Disabilities Act. *15. Nova L. Rev.* 31.

Postol, L., & Kadue, D. (1991). An employer's guide to the Americans with Disabilities Act. *Labor Law J.* 323.

Shaller, E. (1991). 'Reasonable accommodation' under the Americans with Disabilities Act—What does it mean? *16. Employee Relations L. J.* 431.

Shaller, E., & Rosen, D. (1991-1992). A guide to the EEOC's final regulations on the Americans with Disabilities Act. *17. Employee Relations L. J.* 405.

Weirich, C., "Reasonable Accommodation Under the Americans with Disabilities Act," *7. The Labor Lawyer* 27 (1991).

· 9 ·

Responsible and Responsive Rehabilitation Consultation on the ADA

The Importance of Training for Psychologists

Deborah A. Pape and Vilia M. Tarvydas

Many authorities have hastened to hail the Americans with Disabilities Act (ADA) of 1990 as the most far reaching and important legislation to protect the employment rights of persons with disabilities (Adams, 1991; Owen, 1992; Perlman & Kirk, 1991; Hablutzel, Hablutzel, & Gillio, 1992). The scope of its application will no doubt unfold over the upcoming decade, but even the most gross estimates of its impact are stunning. Clearly, the approximately 43 million persons with disabilities who experience a 64–79% unemployment rate (Harris, 1986) remain the most disadvantaged minority group in America today (DeLoach, 1992). The provisions of the ADA are a dramatic attempt to assist in opening "the doors of opportunity for millions of isolated, dependent Americans to become employees, tax-payers and welcome participants in the life of their communities" (Dart, 1990, p.1). This Act took over seven years to develop, and extends equal opportunity in employment protections for persons with disabilities into both public and private sectors, covering an amazing seven million employers (Bowe, 1992). The major involvement of persons with disabilities themselves in this effort and societal recognition of the need to view the massive needs of persons with disabilities from a civil rights perspective have solidified the legitimacy of considering the problems of persons with disabilities from a minority rights perspective. Owen (1992) wrote that the ADA has "smashed the ghetto walls seen by the general public as separating 'the handicapped' from the rest of society" (p. 40).

Many authorities have found this legislative moment to be a critical juncture for rehabilitation professionals to reexamine their understanding of rehabilitation and their preparation to provide services to consumers within

169

the new context created by this paradigm shift. From a traditional clinical perspective, disability has been seen as a problem located within the individual. The minority-group model of disability interprets the problem as located within the social–political environment in which the person with the disability is embedded (Hahn, 1989). Walker (1992) has challenged all rehabilitation professionals to critically reexamine the philosophy and policies of rehabilitation services within the context of the contemporary paradigm shifts. She identified three interrelated camps, the consumers, rehabilitation professionals, and supported employment advocates, and noted that: "What professionals did not see in the traditional rehabilitation paradigm was that they had isolated the problem within the individual rather than considering the context in which the individual was nested" (Walker, 1992, p.15).

Similarly, it is within the context of ADA consultation that psychologists providing rehabilitation services will meet their greatest challenge to reformulate their traditional clinical models of practice. Psychologists have been involved primarily in assessing and treating the problem as if it were located within the person. They have been less involved in addressing the vocational, economic, and social environments in which the client lives. While some attention to the environmental factors in disability has been an early aspect of rehabilitation psychology practice, the mandate of the paradigm shift for those providing consultation is major and unprecedented. Adjustment to this contextual standpoint will involve substantial efforts for psychologists to become versed not only in the technical provisions of the law, but also in the spirit of its intent. New or upgraded psychological knowledge and skills will be necessary to assist persons with disabilities, employers, coworkers, and the rehabilitation team in its full implementation.

Scope of Practice Issues

Authorities have begun to develop an impressive array of potential service needs that the ADA has mandated for both persons with disabilities and employers. A survey of types of ADA services may provide an initial framework for understanding the scope of training demands on individual psychologists. Employers may have need for consultation in determining site accessibility, establishing job descriptions, and the essential and marginal functions of the job. At times this service may be based upon a more specific job analysis (Field & Norton, 1992). In analyzing the suitability of a candidate for a particular job, workers' traits and their needs for specific job accommodations must be determined. A related issue would be an analysis of whether an undue hardship results to the employer if reasonable accommodations were made, or if a direct threat to the employee or others would exist if the candidate assumed the job (Field & Norton, 1992). Other authorities have explored more specialized aspects of this new service arena in an edited text by Hablutzel and McMahon (1992). They reviewed human resource policies for compliance issues in areas such as employee selection and classification, discipline, time off, and salary administration; accommodation of persons with work-related injuries; drug and alcohol testing; AIDS/HIV disease and the ADA; and issues in satisfying persons with disabilities as consumers. Less apparent issues may include the type and extent of needs among the other participants in the equalization of opportunity for employment of the person with a disability—co-workers, direct supervisors, and the employee's family. Another aspect of ADA compliance involves the provision of direct psychosocial services to prepare and support the person with the disability vocationally, psychologically, and socially while undergoing the job search, screening, placement process, and period of adjustment to the new job.

Clearly, the scope of considerations potentially involved in ADA compliance is vast and may call upon many types of expertise. Psychologists interested in providing rehabilitation services with respect to the ADA would do well to consider at least two critical concepts as they go about structuring their scope of ADA practice: the ethical importance of the appropriate training to determine areas of psychologists' competence within their individual scopes of practice; and the interdisciplinary model of rehabilitation service provision. First, competency issues may confront nonrehabilitation psychologists establishing a practice in the area of ADA consultation. Nonrehabilitation psychologists may be approached from a closely allied or customary area of practice, such as in employment testing and evaluation of a job candidate. Typically, as a psychologist from an alternative area of practice moves into increased ADA consultation, there may be a lack of knowledge of the ADA, lack of sophistication regarding the overall context of rehabilitation, a lack of sufficient experience in working with persons with particular disabilities, or unfamiliarity with employer consultation strategies. The psychologist may also be gradually requested to take on other related, but unfamiliar aspects of service, such as the determination of the cognitive demands of a job analysis. As a result of this unplanned process, psychologists may easily find themselves unwittingly operating outside the parameters of their scopes of practice. For example, while rehabilitation psychologists who have master's degrees in rehabilitation counseling may be ideally suited to address employer and vocational concerns in the community environment, they may have a poor grasp of organizational human resources policies or consultation strategies. Conversely, consulting psychologists with strong industrial/organizational psychology backgrounds may be prepared to address the latter issues, but have limited exposure to the analysis of functional limitations of persons with various disabilities and the attitudinal barriers relevant to adjustment on a new job. Obviously, each type of psychologist would need a very differently structured training plan to successfully engage in ADA consultation practice. Several writers have emphasized the ethical requirement that consultants only provide services within the scope of their professional qualifications. They have called for wider utilization of the APA guidelines or specific codes of ethics for consultation to further guide ethical provision of specific consulting services (Robinson & Gross, 1985; Tokunaga, 1984; Gallessich, 1982).

The second aspect of scope of practice to be considered is that most rehabilitation services, including ADA consultation, are provided within an interdisciplinary team context. This concept is salient whether the team members are directly involved or available through indirect consultation. Ethical standards for psychologists have not explicitly considered the obligations to the team and professionals from this perspective, even though it is a time-honored concept within rehabilitation practice (Wright, B.A., 1984; Wright, G.N., 1981). It has been traditional, however, that psychological services be delivered in such a manner that avoids interference with ongoing or pre-existing relationships with other professionals (Keith-Spiegel & Koocher, 1985). It would be incumbent upon psychologists entering into ADA-related practice to inform themselves about the professional disciplines already practicing within this area, such as rehabilitation counseling, vocational evaluation, occupational therapy, physical therapy, rehabilitation engineering, occupational medicine, ergonomics, and speech and language therapy. Persons who are disabled have often had, or are currently receiving services from these professionals. Psychologists might do well to consider drawing upon this base expertise, or establishing a new team partnership as they provide services. This strategy would determine if the best manner in which the unique and specialized expertise areas of a particular psychologist would be complimentary to this constellation of expertise, and would allow for more responsible services. It also would allow a psychologist to provide more in-depth focus on issues the other professionals are less well prepared to address, such as the individualized assessment of and compensation for neuropsychological, behavioral, social, or psychological factors relevant to the job.

The ADA and the Evolution of Rehabilitation Psychology

The advent of the ADA and all its attendant possibilities for psychologists comes at an interesting time in the evolution of rehabilitation psychology. The continued efforts to gain clearer definition for rehabilitation psychology as a particular specialty area of psychology with a specific theory, practice, and training base have yet to reach their ultimate conclusion (Shontz & Wright, 1980; Eisenberg & Jansen, 1983; Jansen, 1986; Morris, 1987a, 1987b). The roles taken by psychologists in a rehabilitation setting may be complicated by the limited "rehabilitation-directedness" of their preparation and experiences. Parker and Chan (1990) investigated these factors in a sample of Directors of Psychology Services in hospitals and specialized settings accredited by the Commission on Accreditation of Rehabilitation Facilities (CARF). They found that clinical psychology was identified by 60% of the respondents as their degree specialty area, with counseling identified by 21% of the subjects.

Rehabilitation psychology degree specialty was noted by only 4 percent. Only 48 percent of all respondents identified themselves as rehabilitation psychologists as defined by the Division of Rehabilitation Psychology (22) brochure of the American Psychological Association (APA). At the level of master's preparation, 53 percent of the respondents had psychology, 12 percent had counseling, 10 percent had "other", and 5 percent had rehabilitation counseling degrees. Parker and Chan (1990) noted that "these data do not enhance a profile of a rehabilitation-directed person" (p.247). The backgrounds of such individuals also would not appear to enhance their image as professionals prepared to address the employment and social environmental environments which constitute such a critical aspect of ADA practice.

In their survey of Division 22 members, Kelley and Schiro-Geist (1992) did find some significant differences in clinical, counseling, and rehabilitation trained respondents in their perceived competency in utilizing various assessment measures, and perceived knowledge of theory within rehabilitation psychology. Clinically trained psychologists saw themselves as more competent in neuropsychological assessment measures than those with either counseling or rehabilitation backgrounds. More counseling and rehabilitation psychology than clinically trained psychologists indicated competency in vocational assessment. In terms of perceived knowledge of rehabilitation psychology, rehabilitation trained respondents indicated a higher level of knowledge than those with counseling or clinical training.

These two studies call attention to the diversity embodied within the background, and perceived competencies of psychologists working within clinical rehabilitation settings. It is also true that rehabilitation psychologists are being sought after in settings such as hospitals, head injury programs, and pain clinics (Parker & Chan, 1990). While many positions are available, it has not been possible to fill them with psychologists trained specifically in rehabilitation, and Morris (1987a) described the tendency for employers to state that "a background in rehabilitation is preferred, but not essential for functioning as a rehabilitation psychologist" (p.1). Most recently, professional psychologists have been noting the increasing opportunities within rehabilitation for psychological services at a time when other avenues are becoming more competitive for psychology. Frank, Gluck, and Buckelew (1990) noted the growth of potential for rehabilitation psychology in inpatient programs, comprehensive outpatient rehabilitation facilities (CORFs), Medicare-covered services, vocational rehabilitation, special education, and managed health care environment. While describing a wide range of possible options for involvement, clearly the emphasis of such observers is on the hospital-based or health care systems in which most rehabilitation psychologists have tended to concentrate their practice. Leung (1990) did a 10-year survey of the positions opportunities in rehabilitation psychology and described the tendency toward an almost exclusive relationship with hospital settings. In fact, Frank, Gluck, and Buckelew (1990) underscored the perceived importance of that point of reference to professional psychology by observing that "indeed, rehabilitation may be the one area in which psychologists can achieve parity rapidly with physicians. Because psychologists fill unique niches in the rehabilitation setting, it is possible that the parity can be achieved with the support and encouragement of physicians" (p. 758). Such a perspective may motivate an influx of psychologists into rehabilitation practice, but provides little promise of an increase of the types of preparation and perspectives needed to make the service model more consistent with the community–focused practice of the vocationally and environmentally grounded ADA–oriented practice. Possibly it is the realization of this gap which has motivated the Rehabilitation Services Administration to structure its request for long-term training grant proposals not simply to address the acknowledged manpower shortage in the field, but to give preference to those programs which emphasize training for vocational and community-based service.

A different interpretation of a rehabilitation psychologist's role might provide a more useful consideration of the functions of a psychologist on a rehabilitation team. Bush (1992) noted that most writings focus on the role of psychologists within medical rehabilitation, almost to the exclusion of psychologists as consultants within vocational rehabilitation. However, Barry and O'Leary (1989) described a professional psychologist on the traumatic brain injury (TBI) rehabilitation team as its pivotal member. Such a professional must have training in neuropsychological assessment, psychotherapeutic intervention, and principles of behavior management. Additional, less traditionally considered skills include abilities in team facilitation, interventions with family systems, application of the scientific method to interventions, and program evaluation. Others have noted the role as a client advocate in the community as an outgrowth of clinical expertise (Rosenthal & Kolpan, 1986). The particular context of this discussion is TBI rehabilitation. However, the model of functioning within the team and community context is helpful in expanding the notions of the roles psychologists must consider in the interdisciplinary, more community-based practice of rehabilitation and ADA consultation services.

Functional Hierarchies for Training

The debate over models for the training of practitioners in the field of rehabilitation has been ongoing for years. As Parker and Chan (1990) stated, "disagreement and confusion appear to exist among educators and practitioners in rehabilitation psychology in defining the knowledge base, roles and functions, training, and experience defining the practice of rehabilitation psychology" (p. 240). Shontz and Wright (1980) articulated the belief that rehabilitation psychology encompasses a distinctive body of theory, research, and problem-solving approaches. Their contention was that the body of knowledge required to practice rehabilitation psychology cannot be gained by merely completing an internship in a rehabilitation setting. Elliot and Gramling (1990), though, have argued that rehabilitation does not constitute a separate specialty and that persons with mental or physical disabilities would be better served by clinical or counseling psychologists trained in traditional psychology, augmented by internship experience. Kelley and Schiro-Geist's (1992) recent study suggests that individuals from each type of doctoral program have unique strengths and contributions to offer the field of rehabilitation. Overall, it should be noted that doctoral level practitioners in rehabilitation will continue to come from many backgrounds and educational bases.

The issues that need to be addressed concretely by all practitioners in the field of rehabilitation at this time is what particular competencies are necessary for rehabilitation psychologists to possess in order to adequately address the issues now arising as a result of the ADA. What role will rehabilitation psychologists play with regard to this important civil rights legislation for persons with disabilities? In addition to rehabilitation psychologists, consulting, counseling, and clinical psychologists will be drawn into consultation practice regarding implementation of the ADA if they work in the area of rehabilitation. As McMahon and Shaw (1992) stated, many rehabilitation professionals have launched themselves into the consulting business armed with only superficial awareness of the needs and concerns of employers, employees, and of the ADA itself.

A Model for Consultative Practice

What follows is the description of a model for consultative practice by psychologists in rehabilitation related to the ADA (see Figure 9.1). This model articulates a hierarchy of functions for psychologists to possess and in which they should be fluent (see Table 9.1).

Table 9.1. Core Knowledge, Principles, and Functions
Related to ADA Consultation

I. Rehabilitation Principles, Knowledge, and Functions

*1. Team facilitation. Providing information to the interdisciplinary rehabilitation team regarding team structure and task; the interrelationship among team member positions; and the roles and responsibilities of each team member in order to improve team performance. Cross-training team members to increase understanding of disciplinary contributions. Being a team leader within the rehabilitation process.

2. Education of clients regarding their rights under federal and state laws. Interpret policies, laws, and regulations to clients and others.

3. Encouragement of participation of the family and/or significant others in the rehabilitation process.

4. Work with advocacy groups to promote rehabilitation programs.

5. Promotion of public awareness and legislative support of rehabilitation programs.

6. Application of the principles of rehabilitation legislation to daily practice.

7. Identification, problem solving, and decision-making regarding ethical issues and dilemmas in rehabilitation.

*8. Identification of psychological, social, cultural, economic, environmental, and physical factors that may impede and facilitate rehabilitation progress. Integration of assessment data to describe functional limitations and strengths for purposes of vocational planning. Counseling clients regarding psychoeducational needs based on assessment information.

*9. Assistance of clients to select jobs consistent with their values, abilities, interests, and functional abilities. Review sources of information with clients (i.e., medical or neuropsychological information) to determine the vocational implications of their functional limitations.

10. Selection of evaluative instruments and techniques according to their appropriateness and usefulness for a particular client. Administration of tests utilizing criteria related to functional limitations, when appropriate. Explore utilization of adjunct techniques to better individualize assessments to the unique needs of clients and in specific environmental conditions of jobs in question.

11. Performance of selected aspects of a job analysis, particularly related to the assessment of psychological and cognitive functioning, as these relate to essential job functions and tasks.

*12. Recommendation of modifications of job tasks or the use of assistive devices to accommodate client's functional limitations, particularly as related to compensation for psychological or cognitive problems.

II. Disability Concepts, Functions, and Knowledge

*1. Knowledge of functional limitations related to various disabling conditions. Providing psychotherapeutic interventions and other assistance necessary to clients in modifying their lifestyles to accommodate functional limitations.

*2. Responding to employers and others regarding biases toward and concerns about persons with disabilities. Addressing cognitive, affective, and social sources of myths about disability and developing strategies at various levels (individual and environmental) to counteract them.

3. Provision of information, assertiveness or social skills training for clients to help them answer other individuals' questions about their disabilities.

*4. Tutoring the individual, his or her family, and others in the individual's network concerning the skills of advocacy.

*5. Counseling with clients to identify emotional reactions to disability. Application of psychological and social theory to develop strategies for rehabilitation interventions.

6. Knowledge regarding cultural and ethnic diversity and disability, and the implications of dual minority status. (i.e., disability with spinal cord injury and being an African-American).

7. Knowledge of psychosocial adjustment models of disability and chronic illness.

III. ADA Knowledge and Functions

*1. Serve as a facilitator/advisor to an ADA Opportunity Task Force Committee in order to build organizational support for compliance activities related to the ADA and develop problem solving within the organization regarding the ADA (McMahon & Shaw, 1992).

*2. Analyze the psychological and cognitive demands of a job (including mnemonic, perceptual, emotional, social, or behavioral components) and work to integrate this information into a complete job analysis. Provide the employer with this information so that an accurate assessment can be made of a person with a disability's abilities to perform the job.

*3. Assist employers in the development of reasonable accommodation methods that go beyond the standard arena of job site modification, job restructuring, etc., and instead involve creative solutions such as: natural support conditions in-house (e.g., co-workers as job trainers; promotion of mentoring relationships), or the use of environmental devices/cues to facilitate adjustment and/or placement (Fabian & Luecking, 1991).

4. Suggest specific devices and adaptive equipment that allows the employer to hire a person with a disability who, with the assistance of the device, can perform the essential functions of a job (e.g., devices that facilitate problem-solving, memory aids such as log books).

*5. Sensitize co-workers and supervisors to interaction, supervision, and working effectively with persons with disabilities. Provide disability awareness and disability etiquette training.

*6. Adapt tests that, when administered to a person with a disability, will accurately reflect the skill or aptitude that is being measured.

*7. Develop intervention strategies that will enable and empower persons with disabilities to obtain employment (e.g., being comfortable suggesting reasonable accommodation options to human resource personnel). These interventions may include psychoeducational strategies such as assertiveness training or stress management.

8. Serve as an expert witness to help in determining if a person's major life activity is substantially limited; if the person has been afforded the opportunities, privileges, and rights to which she or he is entitled related to employment options; and if reasonable accommodations have been made for the person.

*9. Perform an individualized assessment of an individual's present abilities (i.e., cognitive and psychological functioning) to assess their ability to perform the essential functions of a job with or without reasonable accommodations; or to determine whether the individual poses a direct threat to the health and safety of him or herself or others.

*10. Provide adjustment services to a new employer of a person with a disability, to the newly hired employee, or to a recently disabled employee who wishes to remain at his or her job. Address issues related to possible discrimination in the workplace and how to deal with these. Conflict management/resolution or work team building services may be provided.

* First order functions

| **ADA** |
| **Knowledge, Functions** |
| **Disability Concepts** |
| **Functions, Knowledge** |
| **Rehabilitation Principles, Knowledge, Functions** |

Figure 9.1 Conceptual model for consultative practice of
psychologists on ADA.

The functions are highlighted related to first and second order functions to indicate which ones have priority and may need to be addressed through immediate short-term training. The remaining functions may need to be acquired utilizing more long-term training methods.

The model presented here is based on the work by Reagles (1981), who indicated that there exists "a hybrid core of principles, knowledge, and competencies which have emerged in the more than 100 years since rehabilitation came into being because of advances in medical care" (p. 79). The description of functions found in the hierarchy is an elaboration of the list of content areas suggested by the Education and Training Committee of APA's Division of Rehabilitation Psychology (1993) and various competency items from the Rehabilitation Skills Inventory (Wright, Leahy, & Shapson, 1987). The list of functions, knowledge, concepts, and principles in the hierarchy is far from exhaustive; it is specialized in relationship to psychological practice and the ADA. The use of the hierarchy allows practitioners to assess their own competencies and deficits in various areas and subsequently to plan what type of training is needed to "get up to speed" in ADA consultative practice.

Implications for Training

A selected description of both short- and long-term training options is provided to assist the psychologist in planning a personalized continuing education plan to accommodate training needs related to ADA consultation. Such a plan would serve to increase a psychologist's knowledge and skill base in this area of specialized practice. It also would better ensure ethical levels of competence while increasing the presence and credibility of psychologists in ADA service activities.

Short-Term Training Options

1) Psychologists who work in rehabilitation settings will often have access to a professional who would be able to provide them with assistance regarding aspects of the ADA. This professional is a rehabilitation counselor. Rehabilitation counselors, by virtue of their graduate education in psychosocial and vocational rehabilitation, and training in specialized job placement, have an already established knowledge base and competencies in key ADA-relevant topics. Some of the more prominent areas include vocational counseling, vocational assessment, job placement, job analysis, and skills critical to working with employers. In addition, occupational or physical therapists are professionals who could be consulted to determine the more circumscribed aspects of the physical demands of job functions. A mentoring relationship with a rehabilitation counselor will facilitate a psychologist's understanding, not only of this discipline, but also of the concepts that are germane to his/her ADA consultative practice. One of the authors consults with employers on the ADA and often has the rehabilitation counselor working at the institution accompany her during these consultations, with very positive results.

2) Psychologists wishing to practice in rehabilitation must also begin or continue their own sensitivity training regarding the personal and social impact of disability. Specific attention should be devoted to disability etiquette and disability awareness. Use of person-first language in speech and in written communication related to persons with disabilities is imperative.

(See Appendix for additional information.) Participation in disability advocacy groups or disability task forces can be helpful. Attendance at workshops such as accessibility site survey training provided by organizations such as the National Rehabilitation Association or Easter Seal Society can improve the practitioner's awareness.

3) Psychologists should read any of a number of the resources listed at the end of this chapter. Develop an understanding of the concept of functional limitations related to various disabilities (Livneh, 1992). The psychologist is urged to note that a number of functional limitation assessment formats provide limited consideration of emotional, behavioral, and cognitive limitations. These are areas in which the rehabilitation team is likely to rely most heavily upon the consultation of the psychologist. The work of Thomas (1990) is an example of the increased attention the psychologist might place on these areas. Of equal importance is developing an appreciation of the impact of functional limitations on individuals with disabilities. For example, spending a few hours in a wheelchair can be very helpful in understanding the significant societal and architectural barriers that exist for individuals with this functional limitation. Being able to translate an understanding of these complex factors to an employer may become easier, based on such personal experience.

4) Psychologists should take professional continuing education courses that are disability focused. For example, APA offers continuing education home study programs entitled "Psychological Aspects of Serious Illness: Chronic Conditions, Fatal Diseases and Clinical Care"; "Psychological Perspectives on Human Diversity in America"; and "Psychology and Work: Productivity, Change, and Employment" (Call 1-800-374-2721 for brochure). Continuing education programs designed for rehabilitation counselors may also provide useful offerings. Major rehabilitation hospitals or centers with vocational rehabilitation services may provide continuing education programs available to other professionals. Examples of such facilities include the Rehabilitation Institute of Chicago, the National Rehabilitation Hospital (Washington, DC), Sister Kinney Hospital (Minneapolis, MN), and Craig Rehabilitation Hospital (Denver, CO). Rehabilitation counselor educators at local university settings will often be aware of appropriate options.

Long-Term Training Options

1) Doctoral students who are currently involved in training programs can look to rehabilitation counseling departments in their institutions

for guidance. Students should consider taking courses that will develop a breadth and depth of knowledge in this area, if rehabilitation is the area of desired practice. Examples of useful course titles may include: Introduction to Rehabilitation (Counseling); Psychosocial Aspects of Disability; Vocational Evaluation; Medical Aspects of Disability; Career Development; Substance Abuse; Rehabilitation Issues; Ethnicity and Disability; Aging; Ethical Issues in Rehabilitation.

2) The Rehabilitation Psychology Division and the Division of Consulting Psychology within the APA should take leadership roles in developing conference programs, seminars and colloquia in this area of practice. The APA recently jointly sponsored an international conference in Washington, DC on "Stress in the Workplace" with the National Institute of Occupational Safety and Health (NIOSH). This type of cooperative planning, either across divisions or agencies, is necessary to expose psychologists to the diversity of knowledge related to this area of practice.

3) Pursue pre- and post-doctoral internships or practice in such settings as work-hardening programs[1] in medically related or community-based rehabilitation centers, or in disability management programs within industry. The Commission on Accreditation of Rehabilitation Facilities (CARF) requires a psychologist as a member of the team in all accredited work hardening programs. This requirement has created a fertile environment for participation in settings in which a preponderance of rehabilitation services are provided.

Summary

It is essential that psychologists not be intimidated by the Americans with Disabilities Act. It is an important civil rights law. It grew out of an increasing awareness of the need for strengthened public policies to ensure the integration of qualified persons with disabilities into private sector employment (Satcher, 1992). It protects all of us. Should you or anyone you know become disabled in the future, this law will protect you. The law also provides an enormous opportunity for psychologists to expand their practices into the larger community beyond their offices and hospitals. Consultation to the employment community is an area where psychologists can make quite a substantial impact. Occupational therapists, physical therapists, rehabilitation counselors, and attorneys have already begun developing the expertise they are able to offer to this community. Psychologists ought to be responsible and responsive to this need also. They must begin developing a level of expertise that will allow them to make their own important contribution to the implementation of this landmark legislation.

Notes

[1]Work-hardening programs, which are interdisciplinary in nature, use conditioning tasks that are graded to progressively improve the biomechanical, neuromuscular, cardiovascular/metabolic, and psychosocial functioning of the person served in conjunction with real or simulated work activities. Work hardening provides a transition between acute care and return to work while addressing the issues of productivity, safety, physical tolerances, and worker behaviors. Work hardening is a highly structured, goal-oriented, individualized treatment program designed to maximize the person's ability to return to work.

References

Adams, J.E. (1991). Judicial and regulatory interpretation of the employment rights of persons with disabilities. *Journal of Applied Rehabilitation Counseling, 22*(3), 28–46.

Barry, P., & O'Leary, J. (1989). Roles of the psychologist on a traumatic brain injury rehabilitation team. *Rehabilitation Psychology, 34,* 83–90.

Bowe, F.G. (1992). Development of the ADA. In N. Hablutzel & B.T. McMahon (Eds.), *The Americans with Disabilities Act: Access and accommodations* (pp. 3–10). Orlando, FL: Paul M. Deutsch Company.

Bush, D.W. (1992). Consulting psychologists in rehabilitation services. *Rehabilitation Education, 6,* 99–104.

Dart, J. Jr. (1990). ADA: Landmark declaration of equality. *Worklife,* Fall, *3* (3), 1.

DeLoach, C. (1992). Disabling attitudes: When image begets impairment. In N. Hablutzel & B.T. McMahon (Eds.), *The Americans with Disabilities Act: Access and accommodations* (pp. 9–33). Orlando, FL: Paul M. Deutsch Co.

Education and Training Committee—APA Division of Rehabilitation Psychology (22) (1993). *Postdoctoral training in rehabilitation psychology.* Unpublished draft.

Eisenberg, M.G. , & Jansen, M.A. (1983). Rehabilitation psychology: State of the art. In E.L. Pan, T.E. Backer, & C.L. Vash (Eds.), *Annual Review of Rehabilitation* (vol. 3) (pp. 1–31). New York: Springer Publishing Co.

Elliot, T.R., & Gramling, S.E. (1990). Psychologists and rehabilitation: New roles and old training models. *American Psychologist, 45,* 762–765.

Fabian, E.S., & Luecking, R.G. (1991). Doing it the company way: Using internal company supports in the workplace. *Journal of Applied Rehabilitation Counseling, 22,* 32–35.

Field, T.F., & Norton, L.P. (1992). *ADA resource manual for rehabilitation consultants.* Athens, GA: Elliot & Fitzpatrick, Inc.

Frank, R.G., Gluck, J.P., & Buckelew, S.P. (1990). Rehabilitation: Psychology's greatest opportunity? *American Psychologist, 45,* 757–761.

Gallessich, J. (1982). *The profession and practice of consultation.* San Francisco: Jossey-Bass.

Hablutzel, N. , Hablutzel, M.L., & Gillio, V.A. (1992). Legal overview. In N. Hablutzel & B.T. McMahon (Eds.), *The Americans with Disabilities Act: Access and accommodations* (pp. 35–60). Orlando, FL: Paul M. Deutsch Co.

Hahn, H. (1989). Theories and values: Ethics and contrasting perspectives on disability. In B. Duncan & D.E. Woods (Eds.), *Ethical issues in disability and rehabilitation: Report of an international conference* (pp. 101–105). New York: World Rehabilitation Fund.

Harris, L. (1986). Disabled Americans' self-perception: Bringing disabled Americans into the mainstream. (Study 864009). New York: Lou Harris & Associates, Inc.

Jansen, M.A. (1986). Rehabilitation psychology: New directions? Reflections on the profession and the journal. *Rehabilitation Psychology, 31,* 195–197.

Keith-Spiegel, P., & Koocher, G.P. (1985). *Ethics in psychology: Professional standards and cases.* New York: Random House.

Kelley, D.G., & Schiro-Geist, C. (1992). An analysis of rehabilitation psychologists trained in clinical, counseling, and rehabilitation psychology doctoral programs: Recommendations for future training. *Rehabilitation Education, 6,* 67–73.

Leung, P. (1990). Position openings in rehabilitation psychology: A ten-year survey. *Rehabilitation Psychology, 35,* 157–160.

Livneh, H. (1992). A preliminary model for classifying functional limitations. *Rehabilitation Education, 6,* 319–334.

McMahon, B.T., & Shaw, L.R. (1992). Considerations for the rehabilitation consultant. In N. Hablutzel & B.T. McMahon (Eds.), *The Americans with Disabilities Act: Access and accommodations* (pp. 199–211). Orlando, FL: Paul M. Deutsch Company.

Morris, R.J. (1987a). President's message. Wanted: Rehabilitation psychology—Many apply but are many qualified? *Rehabilitation Psychology News, 16*(3), 1–2.

Morris, R.J. (1987b). President's message. Who are we? Where do we come from? Where are we going? *Rehabilitation Psychology News, 15*(2), 1–3.

Owen, M.J. (1992). Consumer perspective on the preparation of rehabilitation professionals: Perplexing paradox or refreshing paradigms. *Journal of Vocational Rehabilitation, 2*(4), 4–11.

Parker, H.J., & Chan, F. (1990). Psychologists in rehabilitation: Preparation and experience. *Rehabilitation Psychology, 35,* 239–247.

Perlman, L.G., & Kirk, F.S. (1991). Key disability and rehabilitation legislation. *Journal of Applied Rehabilitation Counseling, 22*(3), 21–27.

Reagles, K.W. (1981). Perspectives on the proposed merger of rehabilitation organizations. *Journal of Applied Rehabilitation Counseling, 12,* 75–79.

Robinson, S.E., & Gross, D.R. (1985). Ethics of consultation: The Canterville ghost. *The Counseling Psychologist, 3,* 444–465.

Rosenthal, M., & Kolpan, K.I. (1986). Head injury rehabilitation: Psychology issues and roles for the rehabilitation psychologist. *Rehabilitation Psychology, 31,* 37–46.

Satcher, J. (1992). Responding to employer concerns about the ADA and job applicants with disabilities. *Journal of Applied Rehabilitation Counseling, 23,* 37–40.

Shontz, F.C., & Wright, B.A. (1980). The distinctiveness of rehabilitation psychology. *Professional Psychology, 11,* 919–924.

Thomas, S. (1990). *Vocational evaluation and traumatic brain injury: A procedural manual.* Menominee, WI: Materials Development Center.

Tokunaga, H.T. (1984). Ethical issues in consultation: An evaluative review. *Professional Psychology: Research and Practice, 17,* 210–216.

Walker, M.L. (1992). Rehabilitating a philosophy of rehabilitation. *Journal of Vocational Rehabilitation, 2*(4), 12–19.

Wright, B.A. (1984). *Physical disability: A psychosocial approach.* New York: Harper & Row.

Wright, G.N. (1981). *Total rehabilitation.* Boston, MA: Little, Brown & Co.

Wright, G.N., Leahy, M., & Shapson, P. (1987). Rehabilitation skills inventory: Implications of counselor competencies. *Rehabilitation Counseling Bulletin, 31,* 107–118.

The Americans with Disabilities Act

American Medical Association (1992). *The Americans with Disabilities Act: A prescription for compliance.* Chicago: Author.

The Americans with Disabilities Act of 1990, 101, 42 U.S. C. , 12111.

The Americans with Disabilities Act of 1990, 101, 42 U.S. C. , 12112.

To obtain the text of the ADA in alternate formats contact:
American Printing House for the Blind
P. O. Box 6085
Louisville, KY 40206

Dooley-Dickey, K. , & Satcher, J.G. (1991). *A guide to the employment section of the Americans with Disabilities Act of 1990.* Starkville, MD: Mississippi State University, Department of Counselor Education. Federal Register, Vol. 56 No. 144, Friday, July 26, 1991, 35726-35756.

U.S. Chamber of Commerce. (1992). *What business must know about the Americans with Disabilities Act.* Washington, DC: Author. (1-202-463-5533 — Publication #0230).

U.S. Equal Opportunity Commission. (1992). *A technical assistance manual on the employment provisions (Title I) of the Americans with Disabilities Act.* Washington, DC: U.S. Government Printing Office,

U.S. Equal Employment Opportunity Commission and the Department of Justice. (1991). *Americans with Disabilities handbook.* Washington, DC: U.S. Government Printing Office.

Work Fitness Center. (1991). *Americans with Disabilities Act: Turning disability into work ability.* Moline, IL: Author.

Resources for Psychologists on the ADA, Rehabilitation, and Disability Concepts

Recent Publications with Extensive Reference Listings

Field, T.F., & Norton, L.P. (1992). ADA: *Resource manual for rehabilitation consultants.* Athens, GA: Elliott & Fitzpatrick.

Hablutzel, N., & McMahon, B.T. (1992). *The Americans with Disabilities Act: Access and accommodations.* Orlando, FL: Paul M. Deutsch Press.

Rehabilitation Principles

Isenhagen, S. (1988). *Work injury: Management and prevention*. Rockville, MD: Aspen Publishing.

Wright, G.N. (1981). *Total rehabilitation*. Boston: Little, Brown and Co.

U.S. Department of Labor. (1991). *The revised handbook for analyzing jobs*. Indianapolis, IN: JIST Works, Inc. (1-800-648-5478).

Disability Concepts

DeLoach, C. , & Greer, B.G. (1981). *Adjustment to severe physical disability: A metamorphosis*. New York: McGraw-Hill Books.

Falvo, D.R. (1991). *Medical and psychosocial aspects of chronic illness and disability*. Rockville, MD: Aspen Publishing. Co.

Hartke, R.J. (Ed.). (1991). *Psychological aspects of geriatric rehabilitation*. Rockville, MD: Aspen Publishing.

Marinelli, R.P., & Dell Orto, A.E. (Eds.). (1991). *The psychological and social impact of disability* (3rd ed.). New York: Springer Publishing Co.

Vash, C.L. (1981). *The psychology of disability*. New York: Springer Publishing Co.

Wright, B.A. (1983). *Physical disability: A psychosocial approach* (2nd ed.). New York: Harper & Row.

· Appendix ·

PRESIDENT'S COMMITTEE ON
EMPLOYMENT OF PEOPLE WITH DISABILITIES
WASHINGTON, D.C. 20004-1107

FACT SHEET ON:

THE AMERICANS WITH DISABILITIES ACT
PUBLIC LAW 101-336

PURPOSE

The Americans with Disabilities Act prohibits discrimination against people with disabilities in employment, transportation, public accommodation, communications, and activities of state and local government. Telecommunications relay services are established.

EFFECTIVE DATES

The Americans with Disabilities Act was signed into law on July 26, 1990. Provisions of the law become effective at various times ranging from 30 days to 30 years. Here is a summary:

- **Employers** with 25 or more workers, July 26, 1992.

- **Employers** with 15 or more workers, July 26, 1994.

- **State and local Government** activities, January 26, 1992.

- In general, **Public Accommodations** must be in compliance on January 26, 1992.

- **Transportation phase-ins** for accessibility range from 30 days to 30 years. (See details under transportation.)

- **Telecommunication relay services** become effective three years after the effective date of the law.

EMPLOYMENT REQUIREMENTS

Employers, employment agencies, labor organizations and joint labor-management committees must:

- Have non-discriminatory application procedures, qualification standards, and selection criteria and in all other terms and conditions of employment.

- Make reasonable accommodation to the known limitations of a qualified applicant or employee unless to do so would cause an undue hardship.

Exceptions

The bill makes exceptions regarding the employment of a person with a contagious disease, a person who illegally uses drugs or alcohol, employment of someone by a religious entity, and private membership clubs.

TRANSPORTATION
(PUBLICLY AND PRIVATELY OWNED)

- All purchase or lease orders for new buses and rail cars must be for accessible vehicles.

- Paratransit services must be accessible to, and usable by, people with disabilities. The system must provide a level of service equivalent to that provided non-disabled persons. The providing entity must ensure that all persons with disabilities who need the service can use it. The plan must be submitted by January 26, 1992.

- All demand-response service provided to the general public, and privately-funded fixed route service, must purchase accessible vehicles only, unless it can be shown that the service is accessible when viewed in its entirety. However, all new vehicles which carry more than 16 passengers purchased by a privately-funded fixed route service must be accessible.

- Newly-purchased over-the-road coaches purchased after July 26, 1996 must be accessible. In the case of small companies, the effective date is July 26, 1997. The President can extend this for one year further. The bill commissions a three-year study to determine the best way to provide access to over-the-road coaches.

- New bus and rail terminals must be accessible. In altered facilities, the area remodeled must be accessible to the maximum extent feasible. In major structural alterations, a path of travel to the altered area, including restrooms and other services located in the area, must be accessible.

- Key rail stations must be accessible within three years with extensions available up to 20 years (30 years for some rapid or light rail stations). Amtrak stations must be accessible in 20 years.

- Within five years, one rail car per train must be accessible.

PUBLIC ACCOMMODATIONS

Included is any entity licensed to do business with, or serve, the public such as hotels, theaters, restaurants, shopping malls, stores, office buildings and private social service agencies. They must:

- Assure that criteria for eligibility of services do not discriminate. Auxiliary aids and services are required unless they result in an undue burden or fundamentally alter the nature of the goods or services.

- Remove barriers from existing facilities when such removal is readily achievable. If not, alternative methods of making goods and services available must be provided.

- Make altered facilities accessible to the maximum extent feasible. In major structural renovations, a path of travel to the altered area, including restrooms and other services, must be accessible.

- New facilities must be accessible. Generally, other than health-care facilities and multilevel shopping malls, elevators need not be provided in buildings with less than three floors, or less than 3,000 square feet per floor.

STATE AND LOCAL GOVERNMENT

- State or local governments may not discriminate against qualified individuals with disabilities. All government facilities, services, and communications must be accessible consistent with the requirements of section 504 of the Rehabilitation Act of 1973.

TELECOMMUNICATIONS RELAY SERVICES

Within three years after the effective date of the law, phone companies serving the public (interstate and intrastate) must provide TDD relay services for persons with hearing impairments on a 24-hour basis and at no extra charge.

ENFORCEMENT

- The Equal Employment Opportunity Commission enforces regulations covering employment. For information call 1/800/669-3362 Voice. 1/800/800-3302 TDD.

- The Architectural and Transportation Barriers Compliance Board has the responsibility to issue minimum guidelines to ensure that buildings, facilities, and transit vehicles are accessible and usable by people with disabilities. For information call 202/653-7848 Voice/TDD. 1/800/872-2253 Voice/TDD.

- The Department of Transportation enforces regulations governing transit. For information call 202/366-9306 or 4011 Voice. 202/755-7687 or 366-2979 TDD.

- The Federal Communications Commission enforces regulations covering telecommunication services. For information call 202/632-7260 Voice, 202/632-6999 TDD.

- The Department of Justice enforces regulations governing public accommodations and State and local government services. For information call 202/514-0301 Voice, 202/514-0381 or 0383 TDD.

PENALTIES

Administrative remedies and the right to sue in Federal Court are available. Attorney's fees for prevailing parties are available. The U.S. Attorney General can file suits and seek penalties. States can be sued.

ABOUT ACCOMMODATIONS

Generally, they are not expensive. Many work-station adaptations to accommodate a worker with a disability cost little or nothing. From evaluation of data, the Job Accommodation Network, an international information network and consulting resource for accommodating persons with disabilities in the work place, found that 31% of the accommodations suggested cost nothing, 19% cost $50 or less and 70% cost under $500.

When making an accommodation, consult the individual with disability. Also, the Job Accommodation Network can provide **FREE** technical assistance. Phone JAN on 1/800/526-7234 Voice and TDD, 1/800/526-4698 in W. VA. Voice and TDD.

DISABILITY DEFINED

Anyone with a physical or mental impairment substantially limiting one or more major life activities; has a record of such impairment; or is regarded as having such an impairment, is considered a person with a disability.

In terms of employment, the law defines a "qualified individual with a disability" as a person with a disability who can perform the essential functions of the job with or without reasonable accommodation

FOR ADDITIONAL GENERAL INFORMATION

Write to:

President's Committee on Employment of People with Disabilities,
1331 F Street, NW, Washington, D.C. 20004-1107

Phone: 202/376-6200 (voice)
      202/376-6205 (TDD)
      202/376-6219 (FAX)

All public documents produced by the President's Committee on Employment of People with Disabilities are available in alternative formats.

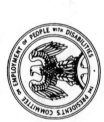

President's Committee on Employment
of People with Disabilities

THE AMERICANS WITH DISABILITIES ACT

REGULATIONS

Copies of ADA Regulations can be obtained as follows:

TITLE I   EMPLOYMENT REGULATIONS

Equal Employment Opportunity Commission
1801 L. Street, N.W.
Washington, DC 20507
(800) 669-4000 (Voice)
(800) 800-3302 (TDD)
(800) 669-3362 (Publications Only)

Alternative formats are available in large print, Braille, electronic file on computer disk, and audio-tape.

TITLE II-A   PUBLIC SERVICES OPERATED BY STATE AND LOCAL GOVERNMENTS

and

TITLE III   PUBLIC ACCOMMODATIONS AND SERVICES OPERATED BY PRIVATE ENTITIES

U.S. Department of Justice
P.O. Box 66118
Washington, DC 20530-6118
(202) 514-0301 (Voice)
(202) 514-0383 (TDD)

Alternative formats are available in large print, Braille, electronic file on computer disk, and audio-tape.

ADA ACCESSIBILITY GUIDELINES

Architectural and Transportation
Barriers Compliance Board
1331 F. Street, N.W.
Suite 1000
Washington, DC 20004-1111
(800) 872-2253 (Voice/TDD)
(202) 272-5434 (Voice)
(202) 272-5449 (TDD)

Alternative formats are available in large
print, Braille, computer disk and cassette
tape.

**All of the above rules are available on the electronic
bulletin board accessed by dialing (202) 514-6193.**

TITLE IV   TELECOMMUNICATIONS RELAY SERVICES FOR
            HEARING-IMPAIRED AND SPEECH-IMPAIRED INDIVIDUALS

Federal Communications Commission
Office of Public Affairs
1919 M Street, N.W.
Room 254
Washington, DC 20554
(202) 632-7260 (Voice)
(202) 632-6999 (TDD)

TRANSPORTATION FOR INDIVIDUALS WITH DISABILITIES

Department of Transportation
400 Seventh Street, S.W.
Room 9315
Washington, DC 20590
(202) 366-4390 (Voice)
(202) 366-1656 (Voice)
(202) 366-4567 (TDD)

Copies of the rule in accessible
formats will be made available upon
request

National Institute on Disability and Rehabilitation Research (NIDRR)
Regional Disability and Business Technical Assistance Centers (DBTACs)

1-800-949-4232 (Voice/TDD)

Your free call will ring through to the NIDRR DBTAC responsible for the region that contains your area code.

I New England
DBTAC
CT, ME, MA, NH, RI, VT

U. of So. Maine- Muskie
Inst. of Public Affairs

145 Newbury St.
Portland, ME 04101
207-874-6535 V/TDD
207-874-6529 Fax

II Northeast
DBTAC
NJ, NY, PR, VI

United Cerebral Palsy
Assoc./NJ

354 So. Broad St.
Trenton, NJ 08608
609-392-4004 609-392-7044 TDD
609-392-3505 Fax

III Mid Atlantic
DBTAC
DE, DC, MD, PA, VA, WV

Endependence Ctr. of No.
Virginia

2111 Wilson Blvd. #400, Arlington, VA 22201
703-525-3268 V/TDD
800-232-4999 703-525-6835 Fax

IV Southeast
DBTAC
AL, FL, GA, KY, MS, NC, SC,
TN

United Cerebral Palsy Assoc.
Inc./Nat. Alliance of Business

1776 Peachtree Rd., #310N
Atlanta, GA 30309
404-888-0022 V/TDD
404-888-9091 Fax

V Great Lakes
DBTAC
IL, IN, MI, MN, OH, WI

U. of Illinois at Chicago/ U.
Affiliated Program

1640 W. Roosevelt Rd., M/C 626
Chicago, IL 60608
312-413-7756 V/TDD   312-413-1326 Fax

VI Southwest
DBTAC
AR, LA, NM, OK, TX

Independent Living Research
Utilization/ The Inst. for
Rehab & research

2323 S. Shepherd St.
Suite 1000 Houston, TX 77019
713-520-0232   713-520-5136 TDD
713-520-5785 Fax

VII Great Plains
DBTAC
IA, KS, NE, MO

U. of Missouri at Columbia

4816 Santana Dr.
Columbia, MO 65203
314-882-3600 V/TDD
314-884-4925 Fax

VIII Rocky Mtn.
DBTAC
CO, MT, ND, SD, UT, WY

Meeting the Challenge, Inc.

3630 Sinton Rd., 103
Colorado Springs, CO 80907-5072
719-444-0252 V/TDD
719-444-0269 Fax

IX Pacific DBTAC
AZ. CA, HI, NV, Pacific Basin

Berkeley Planning Associates

440 Grand Ave., #500
Oakland, CA 94610
510-465-7884
800-949-4232 TDD   510-465-7885 Fax

X Northwest DBTAC
AK, ID, OR, WA

Washington State Gov's
Comm. on Dis. Issues &
Empl.

605 Woodland Square
Loop S E
Olympia, WA 98507-9046
800-949-4ADA V/ TDD 206-438-4116 V/TDD
206-438-4014 Fax

President's Committee on Employment
of People with Disabilities

Telephone Numbers for ADA Technical Assistance

President's Committee on Employment of People with Disabilities
202-376-6200 (Voice) 202-376-6205 (TDD)   202-376-6219 (Fax)

Job Accommodation Network, A Service of the President's Committee
800-526-7234 (Voice/TDD)

Architectural and Transportation Barriers Compliance Board
800-872-2253 (Voice/TDD)   202-272-5434 (Voice) 202-272-5449(TDD)

U.S. Department of Justice
202-514-0301 (Voice)   202-514-0383 (TDD)

U.S. Department of Transportation
202-366-4390 or 1656 (Voice)   202-366-4567 (TDD)

Disability Rights Education and Defense Fund
202-986-0375 (Voice/TDD)   510-644-2555 (Voice) 510-644-2626 (TDD)

Equal Employment Opportunity Commission
800-669-4000 (Voice)   800-669-3302 (TDD)
800-669-3362 Publications only (Voice)

Federal Communications Commission
202-634-1832 (Voice)   202-662-6999 (TDD)

National Association of the Deaf
301-587-1788 (Voice)   301-587-1789 (TDD)

National Association of Protection and Advocacy Systems
202-408-9514 (Voice)   202-408-9521 (TDD)

National Center for Law and the Deaf
202-651-5373 (Voice/TDD)

National Institute on Disability and Rehabilitation Research
202-205-9151 (Voice)   202-205-9136 (TDD)

Project Action - National Easter Seal Society
202-347-3066 (Voice)   202-347-7385 (TDD)

Rehabilitation Services Administration
202-205-9331 (Voice)   202-205-5538 (TDD)

Employer Resources

Programs and Resources for Employers

Employer Incentives/Resources			
Program	**Description**	**Restrictions**	**More Information**
Abledata	Contains more than 15,000 listings of adaptive devices for all disabilities. A consumer referral service that responds with printed reports to requests for information.	Does not make diagnoses.	Abledata 8455 Colesville Rd. #935 Silver Spring, MD 20910 -3319 1-800-346-2742 voice/tdd 301-588-9284 voice/tdd
Disabled Access Credit (Section 44 of the IRS Code)	Encourages small businesses to comply with the Americans with Disabilities Act by allowing a tax credit of up to $5,000 a year.	Expenditures must exceed $250 and may not exceed $10,250. Can only deduct up to 50% of "eligible access expenditures".	Internal Revenue Service
IBM Special Needs Information Referral Center	Conducts database searches in response to specific queries. Will provide resource guides and instructional videotapes upon request.	None	1-800-426-2133 voice 1-800-284-9482 tdd
Job Accommodation Network (JAN)	Free consulting service on available aids, devices and methods for accommodating workers with disabilities.	None	1-800-526-7234 voice/tdd
Job Training and Partnership Act (JTPA)	Customized training or retraining to meet local employer needs.	Employer must hire trainee with intent of permament full-time position.	Private Industry Council (State or Local) Chamber of Commerce City or State government
Special Education Transition and Vocational Education Training Programs	Provides training, placement and on-the-job supervision for youth with disabilities. Can gear training to local employer needs.	Restricted to school-age youth.	Local secondary school authorities.
Supported Employment	A technique for providing on-the-job supervision for an extended time period for workers with severe disabilities.	Employer may be required to help fund the cost of "job coaches".	Local Vocational Rehabilitation Agency or secondary school authorities.

Employer Resources (cont'd)

Program	Description	Restrictions	More Information
Targeted Jobs Tax Credit (TJTC)	Tax credit of 40% of first $6,000 earned per employee provided the employment lasts at least 90 days or 120 hours.	May not claim TJTC and OJT for same wages. Certification must be requested on or before first day of work.	IRS (See Publication #907) State Employment Service Private Industry Council Vocational Rehabilitation (Check State and City government)
Tax Credit on Architectural and Transportation Barrier Removal (Section 190 of the IRS Code)	Tax deduction on up to $15,000 spent to make a workplace more accessible for employees and customers.	Improvements must meet Treasury Department standards.	Internal Revenue Service
Vocational Rehabilitation On-The-Job Training Program	Shared payment of the disabled employee's wages for a limited time on a negotiated schedule.	Worker must be a VR client. Position must be permanent, full-time, pay minimum wage.	Local Vocational Rehabilitation Agency
Windmills (Attitudinal Awareness Training)	Enables employers to build more understanding and acceptance in the workplace.	None	California Governor's Committee for Employment of Disabled Persons 916-323-2545

For Additional General Information

Write to:

President's Committee on Employment
of People with Disabilities
1331 F Street, NW, Washington, DC
20004-1107

Phone: 202-376-6200 (Voice)
202-376-6205 (TDD)
202-376-6219 (FAX)

All public documents produced by the President's
Committee on Employment of People with
Disabilities are available in alternative formats.

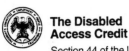

The Disabled Access Credit

Section 44 of the Internal
Revenue Code

P.L. 101-508, The Omnibus Budget Reconciliation Act of 1990, (OBRA '90), contains a new tax incentive to encourage small businesses to comply with the Americans with Disabilities Act (ADA).

The DISABLED ACCESS CREDIT (DAC) is found in Section 11611 of OBRA '90, which establishes Section 44 of the Internal Revenue Code of 1986.

DAC is available to an "eligible small business" and is equal to 50% of the "eligible access expenditures" which do exceed $250.00, but do not exceed $10,250, for a maximum credit of $5,000 a year.

The Credit became effective on the date of enactment of the law, November 5, 1990, and applies to expenditures paid or incurred after that date. It is included as part of the General Business Credit and is subject to the rules of current law which limit the amount of General Business Credit that can be used for any taxable year.

DAC can be carried forward up to 15 years and back for three years, but not back to a taxable year prior to the date of enactment.

An "eligible small business' is "any person" whose gross receipts did not exceed $1,000,000 for the preceding taxable year, or who employed not more than 30 full-time employees during the preceding year. A full-time employee is defined as one who is employed at least 30 hours per week for 20 or more calendar weeks in the taxable year.

In general, all members of a controlled group of corporations will be treated as one person for purposes of credit eligibility, and the dollar limitation among the members of any group will be apportioned by regulation.

In the case of a partnership, the expenditure limitation requirements will apply to the partnership and to each partner. Similar rules will apply to S corporations and their shareholders.

"Eligible access expenditures" are defined as "amounts paid or incurred by an eligible small business for the purpose of enabling small businesses to comply with applicable requirements" of ADA.

Included are expenditures for:

1. removing architectural, communication, physical or transportation barriers which prevent a business from being accessible to, or usable by, individuals with disabilities;

2. providing qualified interpreters or other effective methods of making aurally delivered materials available to individuals with hearing impairments;

3. providing qualified readers, taped texts, and other effective methods of making visually delivered materials available to individuals with visual impairments;

4. acquiring or modifying equipment or devices for individuals with disabilities;

5. providing other similar services, modifications materials or equipment.

All expenditures must be "reasonable" and must meet the standards promulgated by the Internal Revenue Service (IRS) with the concurrence of the Architectural and Transportation Barriers Compliance Board.

Expenses incurred for new construction are not eligible.

For the purposes of DAC, disability is defined exactly as in the Americans with Disabilities Act of 1990.

An eligible small business under Section 44 may deduct the difference between the disabled access credit claimed and the disabled access expenditures incurred, up to $15,000, under Section 190 (discussed on page 4) provided such expenditures are eligible for the Section 190 deduction.

For additional information on the Disabled Access Credit contact a local Internal Revenue Service Office or:

Mark Pitzer, Attorney
Office of Chief Counsel
Internal Revenue Service
1111 Constitution Avenue, N.W.
Washington, DC 20224
202-566-3292

The Architectural and Transportation Barrier Removal Deduction

Section 190 of the
Internal Revenue Code

In 1986, Congress amended Section 190 of the Tax Reform Act to extend permanently the annual $35,000 tax deduction for the removal of architectural and transportation barriers. P.L. 101-508, the Omnibus Budget Reconciliation Act of 1990, amended Section 190 and REDUCED the deduction from $35,000 to $15,000, effective for tax years after 1990,

Under Section 190, businesses may choose to deduct up to $15,000 for making a facility or public transportation vehicle, owned or leased for use in the business, more accessible to and usable by individuals with disabilities. A facility is all or any part of a building, structure, equipment, road, walk, parking lot, or similar property. A public transportation vehicle is a vehicle such as a bus or railroad car, that provides transportation service to the public, or to customers.

The deduction may not be used for expenses incurred for new construction, or for a complete renovation of a facility or public transportation vehicle, or for the normal replacement of depreciable property.

In the case of a partnership, the $15,000 limit applies to the partnership and to each partner.

Amounts in excess of the $15,000 maximum annual deduction can be added to the basis of the property subject to depreciation.

In order for expenses to be deductible, accessibility standards established under the Section 190 Regulations must be met.

For additional information on Section 190, contact a local Internal Revenue Service Office or:

Mark Pitzer, Attorney
Office of Chief Counsel
Internal Revenue Service
1111 Constitution Avenue, N.W.
Washington, DC 20224
202-566-3292

The Targeted Jobs Tax Credit

Section 51 of the
Internal Revenue Code

The Targeted Jobs Tax Credit (TJTC) was originally established in 1977. It was reauthorized through June 30, 1992, by P.L. 102-227, The Tax Extension Act of 1991. Renewal of TJTC awaits congressional action as of this printing.

TJTC offers employers a credit against their tax liability if they hire individuals from nine targeted groups, which include persons with disabilities. The credit applies only to employees hired by a business or a trade, and is not available to employers of maids, chauffeurs or other household employees.

The credit is equal to 40% of the first year wages up to $6,000 per employee, for a maximum credit of $2,444 per employee for the first year of employment.

Employers of disadvantaged summer youth are eligible for a credit of 40% of wages up to $3,000, for a maximum credit of $1,200.

Individuals must be employed by the employer at least 90 days (14 days for summer youth), or have completed at least 120 hours (20 hours for summer youth).

Employers' deductions for wages must be reduced by the amount of the credit.

Individuals with disabilities can contact their local State-Federal Vocational Rehabilitation office to receive a voucher. This is presented to the employer who completes a small portion, and then mails it to the nearest local Employment Service Office. That agency will send back to the employer a certificate which validates the tax credit, and which the employer uses when filing Federal tax forms.

For additional information on TJTC, contact the local State Vocational Rehabilitation Agency or the local Employment Service Office.

GUIDELINES FOR NON-HANDICAPPING LANGUAGE

The use of certain words or phrases can express gender, ethnic or racial bias, either intentionally or unintentionally. The same is true of language referring to persons with disabilities, which in many instances express negative and disparaging attitudes. It is recommended that the word "disability" be used to refer to an attribute of a person, and "handicap" to the <u>source</u> of limitations. Sometimes a disability itself may handicap a person, as when a person with one arm is handicapped in playing the violin. However, when the limitation is environmental, as in the case of attitudinal, legal, and architectural barriers, the disability is <u>not</u> handicapping—the environmental factor is. This distinction is important because the environment is frequently overlooked as a major source of limitation, even when it is far more limiting than the disability. Thus, prejudice handicaps people by denying access to opportunities; inaccessible buildings handicap people who require the use of a ramp.

Use of the terms "non-disabled" or "persons without disabilities" is preferable to the term "normal" when comparing persons with disabilities to others. Usage of the term "normal" makes the unconscious comparison of abnormal, thus stigmatizing those individuals with differences. For example, it is preferable to state "a non-disabled control group" not "a normal control group."

The guiding principle for non-handicapping language is to maintain the <u>integrity of individuals as whole human beings</u> by avoiding language that: (a) implies that a person as a whole is disabled (e.g., disabled person), (b) equates persons with their condition (e.g., epileptics), (c) has superfluous, negative overtones (e.g., stroke victim), or (d) is regarded as a slur (e.g., cripple).

For decades, persons with disabilities have been identified by their disability first, and as a person, second. Often, persons with disabilities are viewed as being afflicted with, or being a victim of a disability. In focusing on the disability, an individual's strengths, abilities, skills and resources are often ignored. In many instances, persons with disabilities are viewed as not having the capacity or right to express their goals and preferences, nor are persons with disabilities seen as resourceful and contributing members of society. Many words and phrases commonly used when discussing persons with disabilities reflects these biases.

Listed below are examples of negative, stereotypical and sometimes offensive words and expressions used when referring to or discussing persons with disabilities. Also listed are examples of preferred language which describes without implying a negative judgement. Even though their connotations may change with time, the rationale behind use of these expressions provides a basis for language re-evaluation. The specific recommendations are not intended to be all-inclusive. The basic principles, however, apply in the formulation of all non-handicapping language.

EXPRESSIONS TO BE AVOIDED	PREFERRED EXPRESSIONS

1. Put people first, not their disability

disabled person	person with (who has) a disability
defective child	child with a congenital disability
	child with a birth impairment
mentally ill person	person with mental illness or psychiatric disability

Preferred expressions avoid the implication that the person as a whole is disabled or defective.

2. Do not label people by their disability

epileptics	individuals with epilepsy
amputee	person with an amputation
paraplegics	individuals with paraplegia
schizophrenics	people who have schizophrenia
the disabled	people with disabilities
the retarded	children with mental retardation
the mentally ill	People with a mental illness or psychiatric disability
the CMI or SPMI	people with long-term or serious and persistent mental illness or psychiatric disabilities

Because the person is not the disability, the two concepts should be separate.

3. Do not over-extend the severity of a disability

the physically disabled	individuals with a physical disability
the learning disabled	children with specific learning disabilities
a retarded adult	adult with mental retardation
chronic mental illness	long-term or persistent mental illness or psychiatric disability

Preferred expressions limit the scope of the disability. Even if a person has a particular physical disability this does not mean that the person is unable to do all physical activities. Similarly, a child with a learning disability does not have difficulty in all areas of learning nor does mental retardation imply retardation in all aspects of development. Chronicity in physical illness often implies a permanent situation, but persons with psychiatric disabilities are able to recover.

4. Do not label persons with disabilities as patients or invalids

These names imply that a person is sick or under a doctor's care. People with disabilities should not be referred to as patients or invalids unless their illness status (if any) is under discussion or unless they are currently residing in a hospital.

5. Use emotionally neutral expressions

stroke victim	individual who had a stroke
afflicted with cerebral palsy	person with cerebral palsy
suffering from multiple sclerosis	people who have multiple sclerosis

Objectionable expressions have excessive, negative overtones and suggest continued helplessness.

6. Emphasize abilities, not limitations

confined to a wheelchair	uses a wheelchair
homebound	child who is taught at home

The person is not confined to a wheelchair but uses it for mobility, nor is a person homebound who is taught or works at home.

7. Avoid offensive expressions

cripple	person who has a limp
deformed	person with a shortened arm
mongoloid	child with Down Syndrome
crazy, paranoid	person with symptoms of mental illness

8. Avoid implying that persons with disabilities are a burden

Discussions regarding the service needs of persons with disabilities and their families often use terms that define the individual as a burden or a problem. Instead, terms that reflect the special needs of these persons are preferable, with a clear recognition of the responsibility of communities to support and include persons with disabilities.

These guidelines were adapted from the American Psychological Association Committee on Disability Issues in Psychology Guidelines for Non-Handicapping Language.

President's Committee on Employment of People with Disabilities

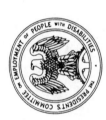

FACT SHEET   SEPTEMBER 1992

EMPLOYMENT ENTRANCE MEDICAL EXAMINATIONS: *Are They Beneficial and Legal?*

Introduction

This fact sheet is addressed to medical examiners, employers (especially human resources personnel) and people with disabilities.

Over the next twenty years there will be a great increase in the hiring of people with disabilities for all kinds of jobs. This is due to two factors: one, a serious shortage of qualified people to fill jobs, particularly in the service industries, which will require use of previously untapped resources of workers; and, two, new legislation which will stimulate businesses to increase job opportunities for people with disabilities.

In order to allay employer concerns regarding the process of hiring persons with disabilities, members of the Medical and Insurance Committee of the President's Committee on Employment of People with Disabilities have developed this fact sheet. It presents the advantages of conducting fair and honest medical examinations, in which the job requirements are fully understood by the examining physician.

People with disabilities are people who can work, in most instances. Pre-existing impairments for which accommodations can be made should be considered as simply limitations and not automatic evidence of inability to perform the job. Medical examinations which serve to match people's capabilities to jobs they can perform will assist both employers and applicants with disabilities. Their widespread use will contribute significantly to increased employment of qualified people with disabilities.

The Issue

Should medical examinations be conducted on persons with disabilities at the time of entering employment? The Americans with Disabilities Act (ADA), PL 101-336, indicates that an employment entrance examination may be carried out provided certain considerations are met by the employer.

The Legislated Conditions

The ADA indicates that "a covered entity may require a medical examination after an offer of employment has been made to a job applicant and prior to the commencement of the employment duties of such applicant," and may condition the offer of employment on the results of the examination provided:

- that all entering employees are examined irrespective of disability - the Equal Employment Opportunity Commission's (EEOC) final regulation governing employment limits this requirement to all entering employees in the "same job category"

- that all findings resulting from the medical history and evaluation are treated as a confidential medical record and are maintained on separate forms and in medical health record files, except that

- supervisors, managers, first-aid/safety personnel, and government officials investigating compliance with the law, may be informed of certain necessary work restrictions, and accommodations, including those suggested by entering employees.

The EEOC regulations do clarify that employers can submit information obtained from entrance examinations to state worker's compensation offices or second injury funds in accordance with state workers' compensation laws. Such information also can be used for insurance purposes consistent with the ADA.

While employers may use as a qualification standard the requirement that an individual not pose a direct threat to the health or safety of the individual or others, that determination must be based on an individualized assessment of the present ability to safely perform essential functions of the job. The assessment must be based on a reasonable medical judgment that relies on the most current medical knowledge and/or the best available objective evidence.

In essence, the post-offer, pre-employment medical examination is an effort to determine if the applicant has the present capacity to accomplish the specific duties of the job, with or without reasonable accommodation, in keeping with the physical, environmental, and psychological demands of the position.

The Rationale

In the past, the examination performed at the time of hire has, for the most part, been used judiciously by employers. While certain employers used the evaluation protocol as a basis for intelligent and beneficial matching of the applicant to the job, it has been perceived that others used the procedure as a device to disqualify persons deemed "undesirable" even though they could perform the essential job functions with or without reasonable accommodation.

Recently, the examination has served many worthy purposes in light of the changing workforce. The medical evaluation has served as a vehicle to introduce the new employee to a health care system or to a preventive medical program. Further, the completion of a pre-placement examination may be necessary to appropriately ensure that a medical condition doesn't preclude satisfactory performance and to offer the benefits listed under the Benefits section, particularly that of identifying reasonable accommodation.

The Benefits

There are numerous reasons for, and benefits from, a pre-placement evaluation. Such an examination can provide the following:

(1) An appropriate pairing of the applicant to the occupational requirements of the job, so that the energy expenditure and the emotional investment in the work completion are attainable and consonant with the individual's capacities.

(2) A basis for determination of needs in the area of reasonable accommodation - sensory aids, special work apparatus or additional devices, relocation of work station, special parking, etc.

(3) An introduction to a health care system which emphasizes wellness and a preventive care ethos, which, if followed can forestall a premature onset of chronic disease or complications of a previously existing disabling disorder or impairment.

(4) A baseline of health status so that future measurements can be used to determine if any job contactants or toxic exposures have proved detrimental to the employee's health.

(5) Discovery of co-existing disease which may be both contagious to others and destructive of one's health.

(6) Knowledge of family health problems so that counsel can be provided, thus reducing periods of employee absence, stress, or lessened productivity.

(7) Provide a basis for liaisoning with employee's supervisor regarding potential emergency situations, e.g. insulin-dependent diabetes mellitus, convulsive disorder, etc.

(8) Compliance with state or local statutory requirements (where mandated) for certain job categories e.g., in primary education, health care, and the like.

(9) A measure of psychological status so that, through referral to counseling sources, future job-related stress can be averted, particularly with applicants who have experienced such problems.

The Examination Content

The usual medical examination performed at the time of employment may include:

(1) A medical history
(2) An employment history to determine possible previous hazardous exposures.
(3) A physical examination which is an organ inventory and appraisal of function
(4) Such laboratory test procedures as indicated by previous or present health status, and exposures inherent in position
(5) Such radiographic examinations as indicated by the history or other evaluation findings
(6) A recommendation, including individualized work restrictions and suggested accommodations, which is forwarded to the hiring authority and which is free of any diagnostic information, and which is used exclusively as an aid in placement.

The pre-placement examination may be performed on the employer's premises, in the occupational health facility (medical department), or may be completed in a consulting health facility external to the company.

The professional conducting the examination must be familiar with the actual functions of the job being offered so that he or she has adequate and appropriate knowledge of the work demands. Any criteria which screen out persons with disabilities must be job-related and consistent with business necessity.

Comment

An examination at the entry into new employment is highly advantageous to the applicant. It provides an appraisal of current health and the opportunity to provide guidance for a safe and healthful work experience. If a disabling condition is present, it can be accommodated to minimize further functional limitations. Meeting the requirements of the ADA is not difficult, for all persons are treated equally and examined equally.

Sources of Additional Information

American College of Occupational and Environmental Medicine, 55 West Seegers Road, Arlington Heights, Illinois, 60005. Telephone (708) 228-6850.

Felton, J.S., "Placement of the Handicapped" in McCunney, Robert J., Chapter 24, *Handbook of Occupational Medicine.* Boston, Little, Brown, 1989.

Felton, J.S., *Occupational Medical Management, A Guide to the Organization and Operation of In-Plant Occupational Health Services.* Boston, Little, Brown, 1989.

Guides to the Evaluation of Permanent Impairment, 3rd Edition, American Medical Association, Chicago, 1988.

President's Committee on Employment of People with Disabilities

1331 F Street, N.W.
Washington, D.C. 20004-1107
202-376-6200 (Voice)
202-376-6205 (TDD)
202-376-6219 (Fax)

All public documents produced by the President's Committee on Employment of People with Disabilities are available in alternative formats.

· Index ·

SP *Springer Publishing Company*

PERSONALITY AND ADVERSITY
Psychospiritual Aspects of Rehabilitation

Carolyn L. Vash, PhD

The author of the acclaimed *Psychology of Disability* draws on her own experiences as a person with severe disabilities to bring us her newest textbook, *Personality and Adversity*. The main theme of this new work centers on adversity as a catalyst for pyschospiritual growth. Using her artistic creativity, the author incorporates ideas from philosophy, religion, and art to provide effective strategies for coping with disabilities.

Contents

1994   296pp   0-8261-8040   hardcover

536 Broadway, New York, NY 10012-3955 • (212) 431-4370 • Fax (212) 941-7842

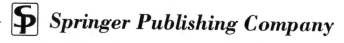 *Springer Publishing Company*

KEY WORDS IN PSYCHOSOCIAL REHABILITATION
A Guide to Contemporary Usage
Myron G. Eisenberg, PhD, Editor

This handy volume presents a comprehensive guide to the current technical usage of key words in rehabilitation. The editor and contributors help to standardize and clarify controversy and confusion in terminology by including core meanings of words and concepts as well as notes on variations in usage. This unique volume also includes an insightful Epilogue on Client-Professional Communication in Rehabilitation.

1993   136pp   0-8261-8320-4   softtcover

DISABILITY IN THE UNITED STATES
A Portrait from National Data
Susan Thompson-Hoffman, MA,
and Inez Fitzgerald Storck, MA, Editors

"...brings together in one sourcebook a national overview of significant, available data on America's disabled population.... Information such as this comes together within the pages of this volume to provide a convenient reference for policymakers, planners, administrators, service providers, and researchers as well as industries that provide products for and hire persons with disabilities."
—From the Foreword
by U.S. Senator **Paul Simon**

Contents: Conceptualizing and Defining Disability • Demographic Characteristics of the Disabled Population • Medical Conditions Associated with Disability • The Need for Assistance in Basic Life Activities • The Education of Disabled Children and Youth • Work Status, Earnings, and Rehabilitation of Persons with Disabilities • Trends in the Incidence and Prevalence of Work Diability • Persons in Institutions and Special Settings • The Economics of Disability • Operating Definitions of Disability: Survey and Administrative Measures

1991 280pp 0-8261-6770-5 hard cover

536 Broadway, New York, NY 10012-3955 • (212) 431-4370 • Fax (212) 941-7842

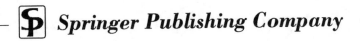

MEDICAL ASPECTS OF DISABILITY
A Handbook for the Rehabilitation Professional

Myron G. Eisenberg, PhD,
Robert L. Glueckauf, PhD, and
Herbert H. Zaretsky, PhD, Editors

A comprehensive text for students preparing for a career in rehabilitation. Covers the medical aspects of disabling conditions including functional presentation and prognosis. Also serves as an authoritative reference guide for the practitioner.

Contents:

Part I. An Introduction to Key Topics and Issues

Comprehensive Rehabilitation: Themes, Models, and Issues • Body Systmes: Overview

Part II. Disabling Conditions: Their Functional Presentation, Treatment, Prognosis, and Psychological and Vocational Implications

Acquired Immune Deficinecy Syndrome (AIDS) and Human Immunodeficiency Virus (HIV) • Alzheimer's Disease • Brain Injury: Trauma and Stroke • Burn Injuries • Cancer • Cardiovascular Disorders • Chronic Pain • Developmental Disabilities: Mental Retardation • Diabetes Mellitus • Epilepsy • Speech, Language, and Hearing Disorders • Hematological Disorders • Obesity • Ostomy Surgeries • Pediatric Disorders: Cerebral Palsy and Spina Bifida • Psychiatric Disabilities • Pulmonary Disorders • Renal Disease • Rheumatic Diseases • Substance Abuse • Visual Impairments

1993   432pp   0-8261-7970-3   hardcover

536 Broadway, New York, NY 10012-3955 • (212) 431-4370 • Fax (212) 941-7842